ETHICAL AND LEGAL ISSUES

For Imaging Professionals

ETHICAL AND LEGAL ISSUES

For Imaging Professionals

DOREEN M. TOWSLEY-COOK, MAE, RT(R)
Former Radiologic Sciences Program Director
Allen Memorial Hospital
Waterloo, IA
Private Educational Consultant
Creative Enterprises Unlimited
Cedar Falls, IA

TERESE A. YOUNG, JD, RT(R), CNMT
Iowa City, IA

Illustrated

Mosby

St. Louis Baltimore Boston Carlsbad Chicago Minneapolis New York Philadelphia Portland
London Milan Sydney Tokyo Toronto

Mosby
Dedicated to Publishing Excellence

A Times Mirror
Company

Publisher: Don Ladig
Executive Editor: Jeanne Rowland
Senior Developmental Editor: Carolyn Kruse
Project Manager: Linda McKinley
Production Editor: Jennifer Furey
Designer: Elizabeth K. Young
Design Coordinator: Renée Duenow
Manufacturing Manager: Debbie LaRocca
Cover Art, Chapter Opener Art, and Text Icon Art: William A. Conklin

CREDITS
Figure 1-1 and Boxes 2-1, 8-1, 8-4, and 8-5 are from Creasia J, Parker B: *Conceptual foundations of professional nursing practice,* ed 2, St Louis, 1996, Mosby.
Box 3-5 is modified from Deloughery GL: *Issues and trends in nursing,* ed 3, St Louis, 1998, Mosby.

Composition by Top Graphics
Lithography/color film by Top Graphics
Printing/binding by R.R. Donnelley & Sons, Inc.

Mosby, Inc.
11830 Westline Industrial Drive
St. Louis, Missouri 63146

Library of Congress Cataloging in Publication Data

Towsley, Doreen.
Ethical and legal issues for imaging professionals / Doreen M. Towsley-Cook, Terese Young.
p. cm.
ISBN 0-8151-2966-1
1. Megnetic resonance imaging—Law and legislation—United States.
2. Magnetic resonance imaging—Moral and ethical aspects.
I. Young, Terese. II. Title
KF2910.R33T69 1998
174'.2—dc21 98-23571
CIP

98 99 00 01 02/ 9 8 7 6 5 4 3 2 1

REVIEWERS

RONALD BECKER, MS,RT(R)
Program Director
Radiography Program
Pennsylvania State University
New Kensington Campus
Pittsburgh, Pennsylvania

LAURA CARWILE, BS, RT(R)(M)(QM)
Program Director, Radiography
Northwestern State University
Shreveport, Louisiana

MEL CHENEY, MR,RT(R)
Director Patient Services
Northwest Arkansas Radiation Therapy Institute
Springdale, Arkansas

BARABARA ENSLEY, RN, CMA-C, MS
Medical Assisting Technology
Haywood Community College
Clyde, North Carolina

SHERI L. HOSTERMAN, RT(R)(CV)
Clinical Coordinator
School of Radiologic Technology
Holy Spirit Hospital
Camp Hill, Pennsylvania

KATHY KIENSTRA, BS,RT(T)
Program Director
Barnes-Jewish Hospital
School of Radiation Therapy Technology
St. Louis, Missouri

CYNTHIA MCCAULEY, MEd, RT(R)
Assistant Director
Department of Radiology
Columbia East Houston Medical Center
Houston, Texas

MARTI MORENO, MS, RT(R), RDMS
Clinical Coordinator, Radiologic Technology Program
Blinn College
Bryan, Texas

JOANN MURRAY, MBA,RT(R)(T)
Program Director
Welborn Cancer Center
School of Radiation Therapy
Evansville, Indiana

SANDRA SALETTA, MBA,RT(R)(M)
Program Director
Northwest Community Hospital
School of Radiologic Technology
Arlington Heights, IL

DONNA SHEHANE, EdD,RT(R)
Associate Professor
Program Director
Radiologic Technology Program
East Tennessee State University
Johnson City, Tennessee

CHERYL THOMPSON, BS,RT(R)
Program Director
Trinity School of Radiography
Trinity Medical Center
Moline, Illinois

JOAN VAN OSTEN, MBA,RT(R)(M)
Program Director
North Iowa Mercy Health Center
School of Radiologic Technology
Mason City, Iowa

In memory of my parents, Rosemary F. and Robert L. Oeth,
who taught me to always do the best job I could but also to find joy along the way.

TERESE A. YOUNG

To the captain of the AT EASE II, Jerry Cook my husband,
whose humor and patience kept me and the boat afloat when I traded my time on the river to be an author.

DOREEN TOWSLEY-COOK

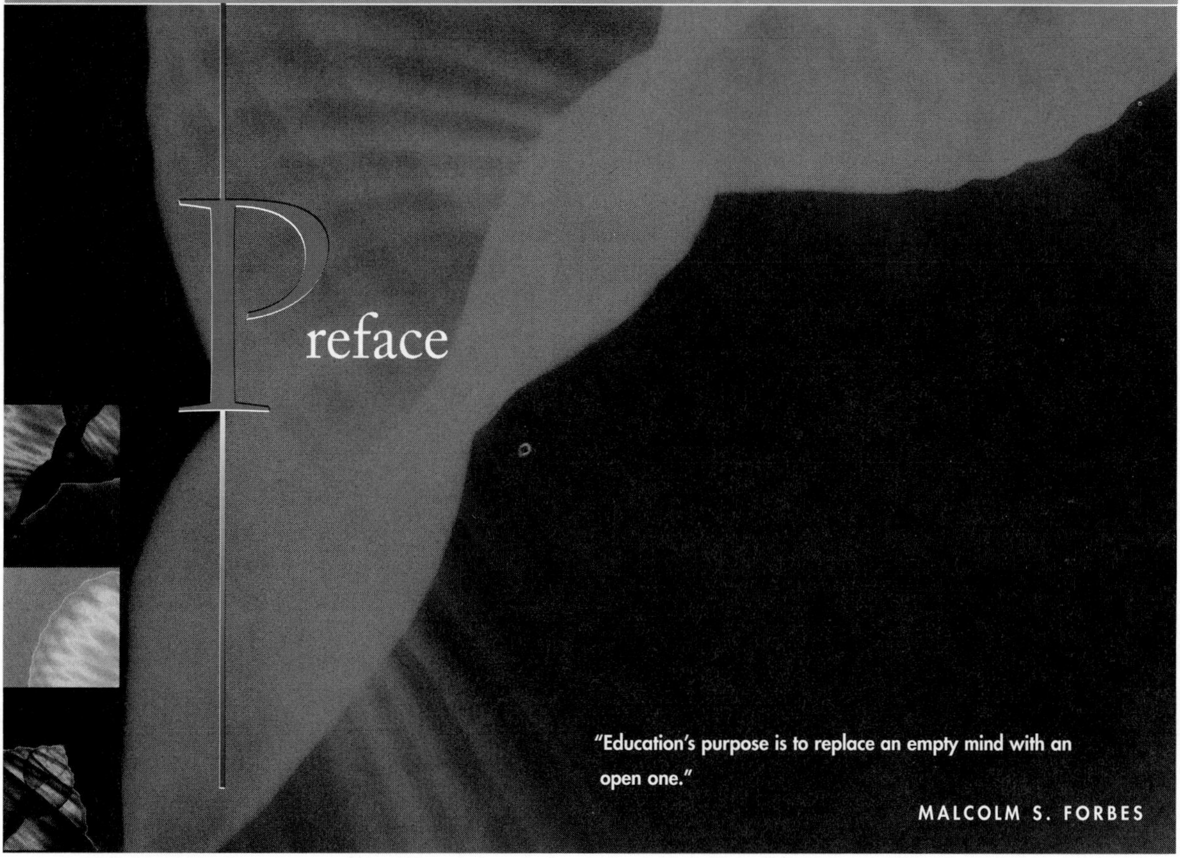

Preface

"Education's purpose is to replace an empty mind with an open one."

MALCOLM S. FORBES

WHY STUDY ETHICS AND LAW?

Many people believe that ethics—including biomedical ethics—is just using good common sense and that medical legal issues are topics to occupy attorneys. Therefore a value system and appropriate behavior should be inherent factors in an imaging professional. Problem solving should just be an exercise in practicality and simply determining the best answer.

Unfortunately, this is not true. Ethical and legal problem solving begin with an awareness of ethical and legal issues in the imaging sciences. It will be the sum of ethical and legal knowledge, common sense, personal values, professional values, practical wisdom, and learned skills that will enable the imaging professional to tackle and solve the problems they will face.

BALANCED COVERAGE OF ETHICS AND LAW

This text provides a good balance of ethical and legal knowledge. It familiarizes the student and the imaging professional with ethical and legal terminology, definitions, methods, and models. Each chapter is divided into two sections: ethical issues and legal issues. Although it was difficult to separate the discussion of ethics and law, they do require individual and specific attention. The study of ethics provides the necessary foundation for technologists to apply professional standards and exercise personal integrity to respond correctly to the ethical challenges they will face. The investigation of legal issues that have an impact on technologists provides a basic understanding of applicable law and equips them with knowledge to allow them to become their own risk managers. After the reader becomes familiar with each topic, problem solving skills in the imaging environment—which frequently presents ethical and legal dilemmas—will be enhanced.

Many questions will be raised throughout the text materials. Some of these, particularly those involving ethical dilemmas, have no completely right or wrong answer, and the student or imaging professional may consider the authors biased. It will be the individual's choice to agree, disagree, question, and pursue solutions appropriate for his or her own conscience. This is the "stuff" of ethics.

This book is being published at a time when health law is changing at a rapid pace. The legal policies discussed reflect the state of the law at the time of publication. Additionally, as is stated many times within the text, the applicable law depends on the particular jurisdiction. Consultation with local counsel is recommended when specific legal issues arise.

LEARNING AIDS

Case studies, imaging scenarios, examples, and relevant current event discussions are used throughout the chapters to enhance the descriptions and explanations of ethical and legal issues. Ethical and legal terminology are set in bold print throughout the text to allow students easy access to important concepts. Profiles from professional radiographers face each chapter opener to pique student interest in real-life application of material. Chapter review questions, scenarios, and critical thinking activities at the conclusion of each chapter provide a variety of opportunities for students to test their knowledge of ethics and law. These activities also serve as valuable tools for building continuing education presentations for imaging professionals.

TEACHING AIDS

An instructor's manual is provided to enhance the teaching of each chapter, designed with the busy instructor and the time-limited class in mind. All activities and discussion questions are designed to be used as separate enhancements to the chapter information. Alternatively, all activities in a particular chapter may be used as time permits or when specific emphasis is required for a particular subject. Features of the manual include the following:

Ethical and legal "What if?" questions for discussion
In-depth discussions of many cases and scenarios used in the text
A variety of activities to use in the classroom
The answer key for the chapter review questions
Suggested audiovisual selections to supplement the chapter information
Transparency masters of key text information

ACKNOWLEDGMENTS

Both authors wish to extend a special thank you to Joyce Barbatti, a most dynamic woman and friend; her helpfulness, timeliness, skills, and ability to do the impossible made the writing of this book a much less difficult task. Joyce is CEO and owner of Barbatti Communications located in Cedar Falls, Iowa. Ms. Young would also like to thank Karla Anderson and Cindy Vest from the University of Iowa Hospitals and Lisa Herman from Drake University Law School Library for their assistance throughout this project.

Ms. Towsley-Cook expresses her thanks to all of her past students who provided her with an environment that continually facilitated her "critical thinking," and to Michelle Manfredi of the University of Northern Iowa's library whose expertise was invaluable.

The goal of this book is to assist in the education of the imaging professional by raising ethical and legal awareness. It is hoped that this awareness will allow the imaging professional to implement critical thinking and problem-solving skills to make appropriate choices in the challenging imaging environment of today and tomorrow.

Terese A. Young
Doreen Towsley-Cook

"Anyone who thinks he knows all the answers isn't up to date on the questions"

FRANK LAWRENCE

CONTENTS

ETHICAL AND LEGAL ISSUES

For Imaging Professionals

ETHICAL AND LEGAL ISSUES FOR IMAGING PROFESSIONALS

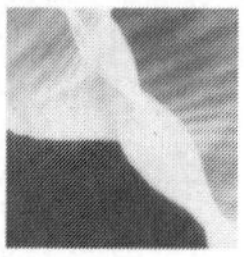

Legal and ethical issues surround me daily in my professional career as I carry out my responsibilities as a lead radiographer and perform specialized radiographic procedures such as intraoperative arteriograms or cryosurgical liver ablations in the operating room. No matter the scenario, legal and ethical concerns influence the way I perform, what I say, and even the way I dress.

When performing any radiographic procedure, I try to maintain focused on the code of ethics that has been set forth by the American Society of Radiologic Technologists (ASRT) and the provisions of the American Registry of Radiologic Technologists (ARRT). Registered radiologic technologists must carry a sense of morality and ethical traits. My choice to become a radiographer was driven by a desire to have technical involvement in the care and treatment of people who are sick and injured. The care given in the operating room and elsewhere implies a sense of responsibility and accountability.

Professional ethics must be adhered to in the operating room and in all other locations in the health care facility. All allied health professionals must practice decorum while in the operating room. Radiologic technologists practicing in the operating room have a commitment to the patient and the surgeon to perform as well as possible in all procedures, whether that be securing the proper view, handing off the proper contrast pharmaceutical, or ensuring the use of the correct technique. They must be alert and conscious of patient rights while maintaining a civil and caring demeanor. We need to treat all persons with the utmost respect and put our personal beliefs aside and work as a united team.

The environment in the operating room provides health care services while maintaining the patient's dignity and meeting specific needs. We all are patient advocates in maintaining quality care. This quality is furthered by assuring patients their right to privacy and confidentiality. As part of the health care team, we act together to make professional decisions and enhance personal accountability.

CHARLES V. CARPEAUX, RT(R)
LEAD RADIOGRAPHER
HARPER HOSPITAL
Detriot, Michigan

CHAPTER 1

Ethical and Legal Foundations

"We don't receive wisdom; we must discover it for ourselves after a journey that no one can take for us or spare us."

MARCEL PROUST

LEARNING OBJECTIVES

- Define *ethics.*
- Identify three types of values that have an impact on the imaging professional's ethical decision making.
- Define *professionalism.*
- List and explain ethical schools of thought and models.
- Explore the schools of thought and models to choose guidelines acceptable to the reader's individual style.
- List the questions involved in the problem-solving framework.
- Define *law* and describe the three foundations from which it is established.
- List the three basic divisions of law and the subdivisions that most frequently have an impact on the imaging professional.
- Identify the three phases of a lawsuit and define the imaging professional's role in each.
- Define *risk management* and the imaging professional's role.
- Identify additional information needed to understand ways to minimize risks effectively.

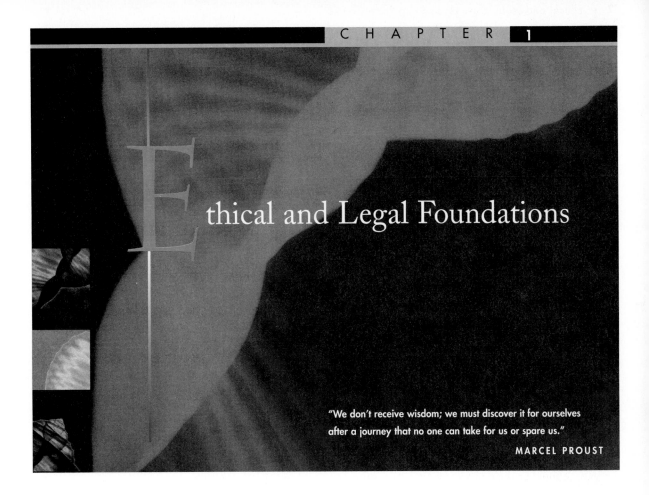

CHAPTER OUTLINE

ETHICAL ISSUES

Imaging professionals face a variety of ethical challenges within medical imaging services. Because of their differing diagnostic applications, individual modalities present specific ethical dilemmas. These dilemmas should be considered challenges and opportunities for growth by imaging professionals. When faced with such challenges, imaging professionals must apply professional standards and exercise personal integrity to respond correctly to the situation. A firm grounding in ethics may help imaging professionals respond positively to the dilemmas they encounter in the workplace.

Ethics may be defined as the system or code of conduct and morals advocated by a particular individual or group. It also is the study of acceptable conduct and moral judgment.[1] Ethics is a system of understanding determinations and motivations based on individual conceptions of right and wrong. It is not determined by strict rules or rigid guidelines, and although it is relatively stable, it can change over time.

ETHICS
Ethics is the system or code of conduct and morals advocated by a particular individual or group.

These descriptions of ethics are broad and general. For the imaging professional, *biomedical ethics* may be defined as the branch of ethics dealing with dilemmas faced by medical professionals, patients, and their families and friends. Biomedical ethics also may be described as guidelines for proper activities and attitudes toward patients and peers. In this case, biomedical ethics suggests a standard of conduct that is expected of members of the profession.

High ethical standards must be the foundation of professional practice to ensure the recognition of the imaging technologist as a competent health care professional: "The development of a code of ethics is one of the identifying steps in the sequence of the transformation of a semiprofession into a profession."[2] Professional codes of ethics help ensure a high standard of practice. A well-designed code lists the principles and rules defining ethically sound practice. It encourages those within the profession to consider the implications of their actions and educates those outside the profession about the sort of care they may expect. A good code of ethics also serves a regulatory function by specifying a standard of conduct by which all members of a profession must abide. Although many certifying bodies in the imaging sciences have developed codes of ethics (see Appendix A), unification remains a challenge. The American Society of Radiologic Technologists (ASRT) Code of Ethics provides consideration of various aspects of the imaging professional's role in health care. These areas include conduct, respect, diversity, technical applications, decision making, aid in diagnosis, radiation protection, ethical conduct, confidentiality, and education.

No code of ethics provides the answers to the dilemmas faced by the imaging professional, nor is a code of ethics merely a set system of conduct. Ethics also is a personal study and investigation. Thus the purpose of a code of ethics is to present a framework for a systematic examination of beliefs that may lead the technologist to an understanding of personal and professional morality and responsibility.

The creation of that framework requires critical thinking. *Critical thinking* has been defined as "purposeful, self-regulatory judgment which results in interpreta-

CRITICAL THINKING
Critical thinking is purposeful, self-regulatory judgment resulting in interpretation, analysis, evaluation, and inference.

tion, analysis, evaluation, and inference."[3] It is an ethical problem-solving tool that allows the imaging professional to perform the following tasks:

1. Adequately interpret and analyze ethical theories and models
2. Evaluate the application of those theories and models to a given situation
3. Plan an appropriate course of action

Critical thinking allows the professional to process personal experience and knowledge and incorporate them into daily decisions. Through critical thinking the professional internalizes and personalizes ethical concepts. Attributes of critical thinkers are listed in Box 1-1.

VALUES

Values determine both personal and professional ethics; therefore ethical questions generally involve conflicts between values. A value is a quality or standard that is desirable or worthy of esteem in itself. Values are expressed in behaviors, language, and the standards of conduct that the imaging professional endorses or tries to maintain.[4] A person's daily experiences influence and guide the expression of values. For example, a professional who attempts to maintain honesty with coworkers and patients has honesty as a personal value.

VALUES
Values are qualities or standards desirable or worthy of esteem in themselves; they are expressed in behaviors, language, and standards of conduct.

Each individual organizes values into a personally meaningful system. The individual's set of beliefs about truth and reality is defined by this system. Thus the imaging professional who values honesty may believe others are honest with him or her because of this personal value.

Imaging professionals prioritize their values, creating a hierarchy. For example, an imaging professional who values honesty also may value privacy to a greater or lesser degree. Depending on the way each of these values ranks within the personal hierarchy, the professional may take several different courses of action when faced

BOX 1-1 ATTRIBUTES OF CRITICAL THINKERS

Able to cut through pretense and fads
Confident and energetic
Courageous
Decisive
Flexible yet systematic
Honest
Imaginative
Intellectually curious and skeptical
Objective
Open to new ideas and respectful of others' views
Persistent
Responsible
Willing to take risks and consider novel ideas

with a dilemma in which both privacy and honesty are involved. This hierarchy may change over time as a result of life experiences and individual reassessment.[5]

Values guide and motivate imaging professionals' decisions and choices, often without their realizing it.[6] Because the motivations and actions of others may be based on different hierarchies and entirely different value systems, awareness of individual values improves communication.

Imaging professionals should use self-analysis to determine their own values before they begin ethical problem solving. Understanding the values of others and recognizing their importance are important steps in ethical decision making. Imaging professionals must recognize that others' values are equally as valid as their own.[7] The three basic groups of values are personal values, cultural values, and professional values.

Personal Values

Personal values are the beliefs and attitudes held by an individual that provide a foundation for behavior and the way the individual experiences life.[7] For example, an imaging professional may personally value timeliness and organization. These values influence the way the imaging professional makes decisions and judgments. Religious convictions, family, political beliefs, education, life experiences, and culture influence the imaging professional's personal values. Each person's values differ.[8]

Cultural Values

Values specific to a people or culture are known as *cultural values.* They also may guide the imaging professional's decision making because they influence opinions about health care. The value of individual choice may be important to an imaging professional from the United States. An imaging professional from an Asian culture may place more emphasis on the value of elderly people than would some professionals from other cultures.[7] Multiculturalism and diversity integrated into the imaging curriculum facilitate discussions of cultural values and their importance to quality imaging services. (See also Chapter 8.) The imaging professional must acknowledge the impact of culture on decision-making processes. Figure 1-1 presents continua of cultural values.

Professional Values

Professional values are the general attributes prized by a professional group.[7] Imaging technologists may learn about their professions' values, standards, and motivations through codes of ethics, formal instruction, and role modeling.

Values in Practice

Values may conflict with one another, with the imaging professional's duties, and with patients' rights. Personal, professional, and cultural values may provide conflicting guidelines.[6] The computed tomography (CT) specialist's value of providing good care for the patient during the examination may conflict with the value of honoring the patient's right to choose, especially if the patient is hesitant to have the examination. The nuclear medicine technologist's value of giving safe doses of

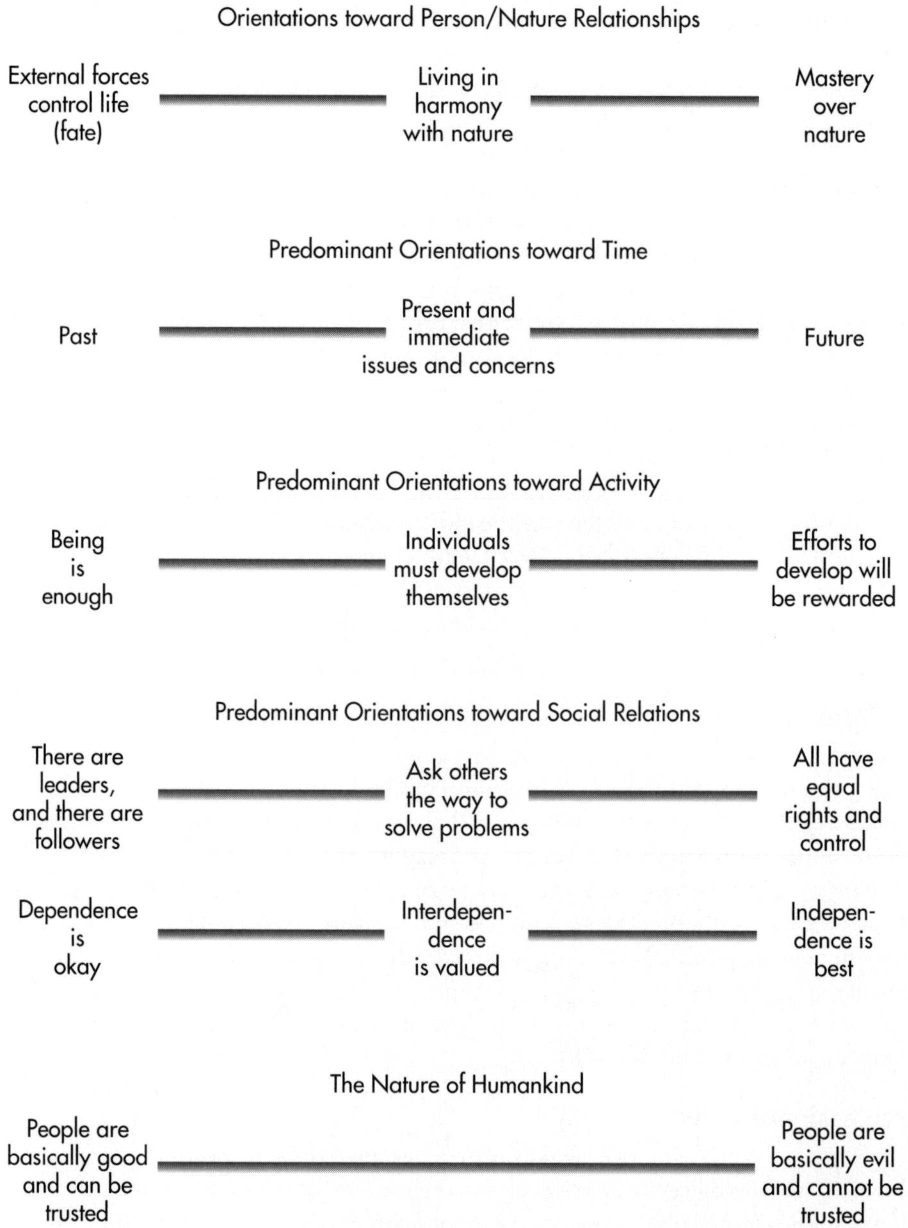
Orientations toward Person/Nature Relationships
External forces control life (fate)
Living in harmony with nature
Mastery over nature
Predominant Orientations toward Time
Past
Present and immediate issues and concerns
Future
Predominant Orientations toward Activity
Being is enough
Individuals must develop themselves
Efforts to develop will be rewarded
Predominant Orientations toward Social Relations
There are leaders, and there are followers
Ask others the way to solve problems
All have equal rights and control
Dependence is okay
Interdependence is valued
Independence is best
The Nature of Humankind
People are basically good and can be trusted
People are basically evil and cannot be trusted

FIGURE 1-1
Continua of cultural values. Ask yourself where you, colleagues, and patients fit on each continuum.

a radionuclide for a therapeutic procedure may conflict with the patient's value of relief from suffering. In each of these situations, imaging professionals must identify the values involved in the decision-making process and determine the most important ones.

PROFESSIONALISM

The imaging professional works in a challenging and changing environment. To respond appropriately to the many potential biomedical ethical dilemmas they will face, imaging professionals must be able to apply the basic concepts of professionalism—an awareness of the conduct, aims, and qualities defining a given profession (Figure 1-2).[9] Familiarity with professional codes of ethics and understanding of ethical schools of thought, patient-professional interaction models, and patient rights prepare imaging professionals to address future ethical dilemmas. When difficult situations arise, they have already thought through the various courses of action and can respond in keeping with their personal standards of ethics.

PROFESSIONALISM
Professionalism is an awareness of the conduct, aims, and qualities defining a given profession, familiarity with professional codes of ethics, and understanding of ethical schools of thought, patient-professional interaction models, and patient rights.

ETHICAL SCHOOLS OF THOUGHT

Ethics may be divided into three broad schools of thought:

1. Consequentialism
2. Deontology
3. Virtue ethics

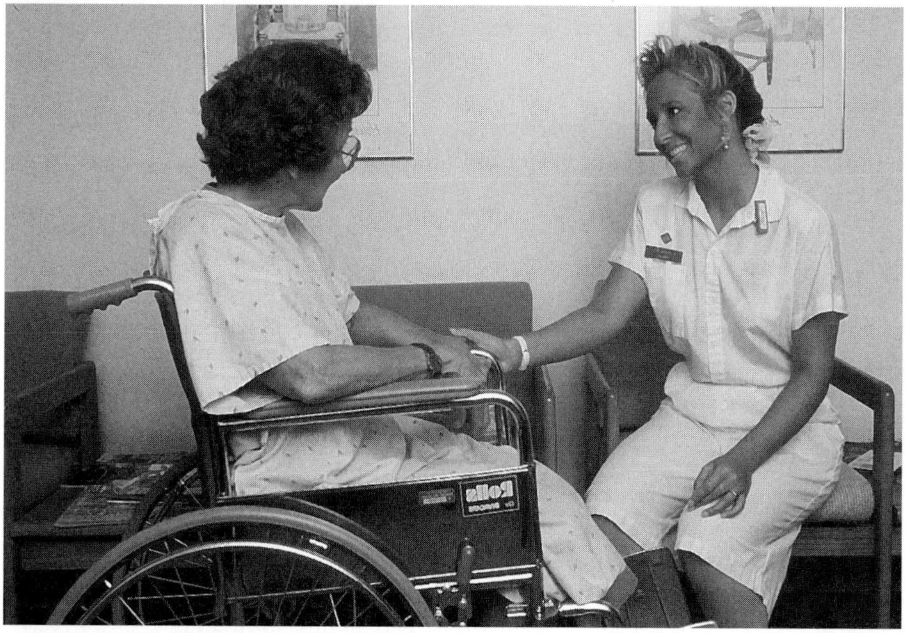

FIGURE 1-2
Professionalism and an awareness of personal standards of ethics are essential for imaging technologists.

Consequentialism, deontology, and virtue ethics are ways of establishing a value hierarchy in ethical decisions. Each school offers different guidelines for ethical problem solving. No one school of thought is better than the others; imaging professionals must choose the one that best serves individual, professional, and institutional goals.

Consequentialism

CONSEQUENTIALISM
Consequentialism is an ethical school of thought in which decisions are based on the consequences or outcomes of a given act; the good of an activity is evaluated based on whether immediate harm is balanced with future benefits.

Consequentialism, or teleology, bases decisions on the consequences or outcomes of a given act. It evaluates the good of an activity by assessing whether immediate harm is balanced with future benefit. For example, a patient with cancer undergoing radiation therapy may experience some discomfort now, but the palliation or cure of the cancer is the desired beneficial consequence of the therapy. Consequentialism advocates providing the greatest good for the greatest number.

Within a teleologic framework, an imaging technologist assisting in triage for radioactive spill trauma patients would assign services to the most critically injured patient last to serve a greater number of less-injured patients. Is this a reasonable philosophy for health care providers? In what way would an imaging director using consequentialist ethics determine ways to cut staffing in a department?

Deontology

DEONTOLOGY
Deontology is an ethical school of thought that bases decision making on individual motives and morals rather than consequences and examines the significance of actions themselves. Deontologic problem solving uses personal rules of right and wrong derived from individual actions, relationships of all kinds, and society.

Deontology bases decision making on individual motives and morals rather than consequences. It is therefore the opposite of teleology. Deontology examines the significance of actions themselves. For example, members of certain religious groups refuse blood transfusions because they feel the act is morally wrong. Although they may be concerned about the consequences of this refusal, they are making the choice based on their religious beliefs regarding blood transfusions. Personal rules of right and wrong derived from individual actions, relationships of all kinds, and society are used for reasoning and problem solving in the deontologic school of thought.

Drawing from the previous example, would the imaging technologist find deontology any more useful in decision making regarding triage for victims of a radioactive spill? Can absolute rights and wrongs in triage be determined? In what way would an imaging director using deontologic ethics determine ways to reduce staff? Should the moral significance of each individual be considered in department restructuring?

Virtue Ethics

VIRTUE ETHICS
Virtue ethics is a new ethical school of thought that focuses on the use of practical wisdom for emotional and intellectual problem solving. It incorporates elements of teleology and deontology to provide a more holistic approach to solving ethical dilemmas.

Virtue ethics is a relatively new school of thought. It focuses on the use of practical wisdom for emotional and intellectual problem solving. Virtue ethics incorporates elements of teleology and deontology to provide a more holistic approach to solving ethical dilemmas. Careful analysis and consideration of consequences, rules established by society, and short-term effects play significant roles in decision making in virtue ethics.

Virtue ethics lends itself to many situations in which imaging professionals may become involved. For instance, an imaging technologist assisting in triage needs to recognize the significance of each individual and the way triage decisions affect the family and friends of injured persons. However, the technologist also works under time constraints and must understand that victims suffer from varying degrees of trauma. A department manager should understand the way staffing decisions will change lives and directly affect the quality and type of imaging services available through the department, but also must be aware of the cost and resources necessary to provide quality imaging services.

ETHICAL MODELS

Models for ethical decision making in health care broadly describe different types of interactions with patients. They provide frameworks for understanding expectations and responsibilities (Table 1-1). Individual health care professionals must choose the model or models they feel are appropriate. Some models may work in certain situations and not in others (Figure 1-3). All the models may be applied to any of the ethical schools of thought presented in the previous section.

TABLE 1-1 ETHICAL MODELS

Model	Precept
Engineering	Provider views patient as condition or procedure
Paternal/Priestly	Provider thinks he or she knows what is best for patients
Collegial	Mutual cooperation between provider and patient
Contractual	Business relationship where provider and patient both have obligations, rights, and responsibilities
Covenantal	Agreement between provider and patient grounded on traditional values

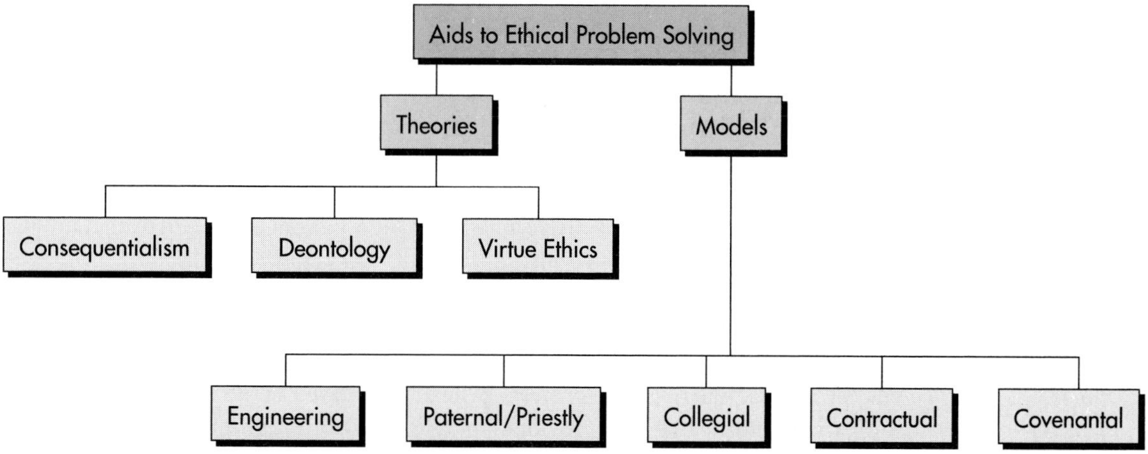

FIGURE 1-3
Aids to ethical problem solving.

Engineering Model

The engineering model identifies the health care provider as a scientist concerned with facts and defines the patient as a condition or procedure, not a person. A health care professional using the engineering model tends to view the patient as a collection of body systems, instead of as a whole. Under this model a diagnostic imaging technologist considers the patient a gastrointestinal (GI) or skull series, not an anxious human patient. A vascular imaging professional using the engineering model believes that primary importance should be placed on the circulatory system, not on the patient's emotional or psychologic needs.

Paternal or Priestly Model

The paternal or priestly model casts the care giver in the omniscient, paternalistic role of making decisions *for* patients rather than *with* patients. The magnetic resonance technologist who powerfully urges a feeble 90-year-old person on the table when the patient explains that he or she cannot make the move is exhibiting paternalism. So is the imaging professional who dismisses the needs of patients who want to know more about procedures by telling them not to worry, that everything will be fine. Those who subscribe to the priestly model generally believe they know best and tend to discount the patient's feelings.

Collegial Model

The collegial model describes a more cooperative method of providing health care for the patient. It involves sharing, trust, and the pursuit of common goals. An imaging professional who takes time to get to know the patient and works with the patient to reach a mutual understanding is working within the collegial model. This model may be helpful in addressing patients' emotional needs and engaging their cooperation. However, it requires the health care professional to have enough time to spend with the patient.

Contractual Model

The contractual model defines health care as a business relationship between the provider and patient. A contractual arrangement serves as the guideline for decision making and provision of services. That is, the patient and provider are seen as parties to a contract in which both sides have obligations, rights, and responsibilities. This model is exemplified in the informed consent process. The imaging professional who explains an invasive procedure to a patient is involved in the contractual process.

Covenantal Model

The covenantal model recognizes that many areas of health care are not always covered by a terse, businesslike contract. Instead, it is based on an agreement between the patient and health care provider, an agreement often grounded on traditional values and goals. These include trust in the professional's integrity and confidence that the professional has the patient's best interests in mind. Many imaging procedures require the patient to trust in the radiographer's competence and professionalism. Therefore the model often used combines the covenantal and contractual models to build a business relationship and implement shared goals and values. The ability to trust often depends on previous experiences with health care procedures. A patient experiencing a difficult pregnancy may trust the sonographer's skills based on values inherent in the covenantal model. Similarly, an accident patient may request to be taken to a specific hospital because of previous satisfaction with services received in its imaging department.

PATIENTS' RIGHTS

Patients' rights are among the most important of the issues involved in biomedical ethics, influencing almost every aspect of the professional's ethical considerations. The American Hospital Association (AHA) has recognized the importance of patients' rights and published *A Patient's Bill of Rights* (Box 1-2).

Patient awareness of individual rights and needs and availability of the various imaging techniques provides both opportunities and complications for the imaging professional. However, quality imaging is facilitated by patient knowledge and participation. The patient's role should include active participation in health care based on accurate information.

BOX 1-2 A PATIENT'S BILL OF RIGHTS

1. The patient has the right to considerate and respectful care.
2. The patient has the right to and is encouraged to obtain from physicians and other direct caregivers relevant, current, and understandable information concerning diagnosis, treatment, and prognosis.

   Except in emergencies when the patient lacks decision-making capacity and the need for treatment is urgent, the patient is entitled to the opportunity to discuss and request information related to the specific procedures and/or treatments, the risks involved, the possible length of recuperation, and the medically reasonable alternatives and their accompanying risks and benefits.

   Patients have the right to know the identity of physicians, nurses, and others involved in their care, as well as when those involved are students, residents, or other trainees. The patient also has the right to know the immediate and long-term financial implications of treatment choices, insofar as they are known.
3. The patient has the right to make decisions about the plan of care prior to and during the course of treatment and to refuse a recommended treatment or plan of care to the extent permitted by law and hospital policy and to be informed of the medical consequences of this action. In case of such refusal, the patient is entitled to other appropriate care and services that the hospital provides or transfers to another hospital. The hospital should notify patients of any policy that might affect patient choice within the institution.
4. The patient has the right to have an advance directive (such as a living will, health care proxy, or durable power of attorney for health care) concerning treatment or designating a surrogate decision maker with

Continued

BOX 1-2 A PATIENT'S BILL OF RIGHTS—cont'd

the expectation that the hospital will honor the intent of that directive to the extent permitted by law and hospital policy.

Health care institutions must advise patients of their rights under state law and hospital policy to make informed medical choices, ask if the patient has an advance directive, and include that information in patient records. The patient has the right to timely information about hospital policy that may limit its ability to implement fully a legally valid advance directive.

5. The patient has the right to every consideration of privacy. Case discussion, consultation, examination, and treatment should be conducted so as to protect each patient's privacy.
6. The patient has the right to expect that all communications and records pertaining to his/her care will be treated as confidential by the hospital, except in cases such as suspected abuse and public health hazards when reporting is permitted or required by law. The patient has the right to expect that the hospital will emphasize the confidentiality of this information when it releases it to any other parties entitled to review information in these records.
7. The patient has the right to review the records pertaining to his/her medical care and to have the information explained or interpreted as necessary, except when restricted by law.
8. The patient has the right to expect that, within its capacity and policies, a hospital will make reasonable response to the request of a patient for appropriate and medically indicated care and services. The hospital must provide evaluation, service, and/or referral as indicated by the urgency of the case. When medically appropriate and legally permissible, or when a patient has so requested, a patient may be transferred to another facility. The institution to which the patient is to be transferred must first have accepted the patient for transfer. The patient must also have the benefit of complete information and explanation concerning the need for, risks, benefits, and alternatives to such a transfer.
9. The patient has the right to ask and be informed of the existence of business relationships among the hospital, educational institution, and other health care providers, or payers that may influence the patient's treatment and care.
10. The patient has the right to consent to or decline to participate in proposed research studies or human experimentation affecting care and treatment or requiring direct patient involvement, and to have those studies fully explained prior to consent. A patient who declines to participate in research or experimentation is entitled to the most effective care that the hospital can otherwise provide.
11. The patient has the right to expect reasonable continuity of care when appropriate and to be informed by physicians and other caregivers of available and realistic patient care options when hospital care is no longer appropriate.
12. The patient has the right to be informed of hospital policies and practices that relate to patient care, treatment, and responsibilities. The patient has the right to be informed of available resources for resolving disputes, grievances, and conflicts, such as ethics committees, patient representatives, or other mechanisms available in the institution. The patient has the right to be informed of the hospital's charges for services and available payment methods.

From American Hospital Association: *A patient's bill of rights,* Chicago, 1992, Author.

CASE STUDY ANALYSIS FOR ETHICAL PROBLEM SOLVING

Four questions may be asked to provide a framework for case study analysis and aid the health care professional considering ethical problems:[7]

1. What is the context in which the ethical problem has occurred?
2. What is the significance of the values involved in the problem?
3. What is the meaning of the problem for all the parties involved?
4. What should be done to remedy the problem?

What Is the Context in Which the Ethical Problem Has Occurred?

With contextual information, the health care professional may discover the way the problem arose, learn the various sides to the problem, and begin to understand the values of the parties. Determining the context of the problem requires the gathering of factual and value information relevant to the conflict. The professional must listen to all aspects of the story to create a complete picture.

What Is the Significance of the Values Involved in the Problem?

The resolution of most conflicts requires compromise on the parts of those involved. The goal of the imaging professional involved in an ethical conflict should be to help individuals prioritize their values to preserve those most important to the issue. The professional must understand which values may be subordinated by the parties at the cost of the least harm. To do this, the professional must determine the significance of all values involved.

What Is the Meaning of the Problem for All the Parties Involved?

Ethical problems have a history and context that render them significant or insignificant to the parties involved. The imaging professional needs to discover some of that context to determine the significance of the problem for all the involved parties. In answering this question the professional may discover the roots of recurring value conflicts and be able to aid in the formation of a policy to avoid future difficulties.

What Should Be Done to Remedy the Problem?

Using information gathered and processed, the professional should be able to offer a variety of ways to resolve the conflict. The involved parties may wish to explore several options before coming to a decision. Imaging professionals should keep in mind that although some options might be ethically permissible, they may not support the values of those involved. Other options (such as assisted suicide or abortion) might be ethically permissible for one party but not for another.[7]

IMAGING SCENARIO

The director of radiology services received a memo from the institution's chief executive officer (CEO) concerning a patient complaint. He began the investigation by listening to all the parties involved and remained objective while visualizing the overall situation. With this approach, he realized the complaint arose from a difference in cultural values. These cultural differences caused confusion and emotional discomfort to the patient and involved issues of being touched, privacy, and communication.

The female patient, who spoke little English, had been scheduled for a mammogram, which was to be performed by a male technologist. Because English was not her primary language and because she was uncomfortable being undressed with a man touching her, the patient became upset and left without her examination. On questioning, the mammographer reported that he had tried his best to explain the procedure to the patient and that he had been pleasant and considerate. Each person involved in the situation saw the problem from a different perspective.

The significance of this situation for the patient was the emotional trauma involved and the lack of completion of the examination. The mammographer failed in completing the procedure. The director of radiologic services was advised by the CEO that mammography is heavily marketed and these types of situations should not happen and are not to happen in the future. How best could the situation be resolved and include recognition of all the parties' values?

The director first interviewed persons from varying cultural backgrounds and made himself more knowledgeable. He then provided a brainstorming session for radiology personnel and asked them to compile a list of possible solutions. One solution was to initiate focus groups that included community members from a variety of cultural backgrounds. The patient was invited and then participated in a focus group to work out solutions to situations such as the one she had experienced. After the many solutions and alternatives were evaluated, several were implemented at different levels, including educational activities within the department and the development of a department procedure and policy to promote recognition of all patients' cultural values in future situations.

LEGAL ISSUES

Imaging technologists face many legal issues in addition to the ethical dilemmas they encounter. Although they cannot be expected to have a thorough understanding of all legal issues, they should have a basic knowledge of law, the legal system, the legal issues they are most likely to encounter, the legal facilities of the institution, and institutional regulations regarding the patient care they provide. An understanding of other legal matters that influence the professional life of the technologist (e.g., student rights, diversity issues, employee-management relations, whistle-blowing) also is important. These matters are discussed thoroughly in later chapters. Imaging technologists should begin their exploration of legal implications for their practices with a broad overview of the law and some of its components, especially the lawsuit and the function of risk management. Specific legal issues faced by technologists and their facilities that influence patient care are discussed more thoroughly in Chapters 2, 3, and 4. Methods to decrease the risk of litigation also are provided in these chapters.

THE LAW

The law is a body of rules of action or conduct prescribed by controlling authority and having binding legal force.[10]

THE LAW
The law is a body of rules of action or conduct prescribed by controlling authority and having binding legal force. Its basis is in common law from England but has been molded by statutes and judicial decisions since the birth of the United States.

The basis for the controlling authority of the law in the United States includes common law from England but has been molded by statutes and judicial decisions (case law) since the birth of the United States (Figure 1-4).

The "common law," which forms the basis for the current law in 49 of the 50 states, includes all the statutory and case law background of England and the American Colonies before the American Revolution.[11] This common law encompasses principles and rules that derive their authority solely from ancient usages and customs or judgments and decrees of courts supporting those usages and customs.[10] Louisiana provides the exception to English common law forming the basis for current law. Louisiana's law is based on Roman law through the French Revolution and the Napoleonic Code.

Legislation, as provided for in the Constitution of the United States, includes all the laws or statutes put into place by the elected officials in federal, state, city, and county governments. Judicial decisions may interpret the statutes and therefore further refine their application. Judicial decisions may reinforce common law principles or change them to match the changes in society.

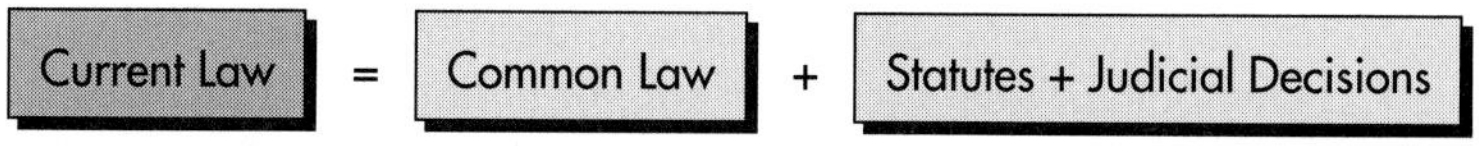

FIGURE 1-4
Sources of current law.

COMMON LAW
Common law encompasses principles and rules based on ancient usages and customs.

Common Law

The following example regarding the origins of the tort of negligence may help to illustrate the common law basis of our current law system. The tort of negligence had its origins in the liability of those who professed to be competent in certain "public" callings. In England and the colonies, a carrier, an innkeeper, a blacksmith, or a surgeon was regarded as holding himself out to the public as one in whom people should have confidence. This act of holding themselves out as knowledgeable in their field created an obligation to give proper service. If such service was not delivered through their personal fault, they might be held liable for any damage or injury caused.

This imposition of a duty of care based on the special position of these professionals and the possibility of liability if that duty were not performed correctly was based on custom. Ancient judicial decisions imposed liability based on this custom. Thus common law regarding negligence was established through custom and judicial decisions supporting that custom.

The current law regarding negligence, which is discussed thoroughly in Chapter 2, originated from this same custom. Negligence can be found under current law only if a duty is owed, that duty is breached, and demonstrable harm has resulted from the breach.

STATUTORY LAW
Statutory law includes all laws enacted by federal, state, city, and county governments.

LEGISLATION
Legislation is all the laws and statutes put into place by elected officials in federal, state, city, and county governments.

Statutes and Judicial Decisions

Continuing the example of negligence may help to illustrate the role statutes and judicial decisions play in current law. Negligence can be found only if a duty exists. This duty can be imposed in several ways. A statute may create such a duty. For example, in Iowa a statute lists the risks that must be disclosed by a physician to obtain informed consent from a patient. The statute has established a duty to disclose those risks before performing the procedure. Judicial decisions that interpret the statutes may further refine the details surrounding physician disclosure.

In a state in which no such statute exists or the statute is not specific, the obligation to disclose risks still exists but has a different basis. Previous judicial decisions (or precedents) in a state's courts form the basis for the duty of physicians in that state. The reasoning on which those decisions are based may well be common law principles that have been adapted to meet the changes in society.

JUDICIAL DECISIONS
Judicial decisions are previous cases that either interpret statutes or adopt and adapt common law principles.

For example, some states have adopted, through judicial decisions, the standard that a physician must disclose to a patient information that a reasonable medical practitioner similarly situated would disclose. This is called the *physician-based standard.*[12] Other states have adopted the reasonable patient standard, which means that the physician must disclose information that a reasonable patient needs to make an informed decision.[13]

Very simplistically, current law is a product of common law, statutory law, and judicial decisions. However, as is evident from these examples, current law can vary depending on the jurisdiction. Additionally, although courts often look to decisions from other jurisdictions for guidance, they are not bound to follow those decisions. Moreover, the law can change as society changes. Therefore, imaging professionals should learn the current law in their jurisdictions.

Administrative, criminal, and civil law are components of the legal system that have an impact on the medical imaging sciences. Administrative law determines the

BOX 1-3 BRANCHES OF THE LAW

Administrative law—Deals with licensing and regulation
Penalties for violation can include suspension and revocation of license
Criminal law—Addresses wrongs against the state
Penalties for violation can include fines, restitution, community service, and incarceration
Civil law—Addresses wrongs committed by one party harming another
Penalties for violation can include monetary damages to compensate for loss and to punish

IMAGING SCENARIO

An elderly patient comes to the imaging department for lumbar spine films. The patient attempts to be cooperative but because of pain is unable to lie flat on the imaging table and refuses the examination. The imaging technologist assures the patient she will be able to lie flat and assists her to lie down against her will.

The patient complains to her son, an attorney, about her treatment, and he contacts protective services to investigate. As a result of the investigation, criminal battery charges are pending against the technologist. Additionally, the patient has filed a civil lawsuit against the technologist and the hospital. The suit alleges medical malpractice based on the hiring of the technologist, the negligence of the technologist, and the failure to train and supervise the technologist properly. Protective services has brought the investigation and charges to the attention of the regulatory division of the State Public Health Department, and they are investigating the incident.

licensing and regulation of the practice of imaging professionals and regulates some employer-employee relations. Criminal law seeks to redress wrongs against the state. Civil law attempts to compensate for wrongs committed by one party resulting in harm to another party (Box 1-3). The same set of circumstances may be the basis of both a civil and criminal case.

Each branch of law has separate and distinct penalties. For example, the imaging scenario above resulted in all of the following: an administrative action involving the technologist's license to practice; a criminal charge of battery possibly involving incarceration; and a civil lawsuit alleging medical malpractice, which may entail the paying of monetary damages from the hospital's insurance company.

Lawsuits involving the medical imaging sciences generally are brought under tort law, a subdivision of civil law. A tort action is filed to recover damages for personal injury or property damage occurring from negligent conduct or intentional misconduct.[14] The types of torts that could possibly be encountered by imaging professionals include assault, battery, false imprisonment, defamation, negligence, lack of informed consent, and breach of patient confidentiality. The tort most often encountered by imaging professionals is negligence. Subsequent chapters explain torts in

TABLE 1-2 THE PHASES OF A LAWSUIT

Phase	Action
Pleading phase	Complaint lodged Answer given
Discovery phase	Facts are sought in two ways: Written questions (interrogatories) Oral questions (deposition)
Trial Decision	Presentation of facts to judge or jury

detail. Imaging professionals must have a basic understanding of the elements of torts, strategies to protect themselves and their facilities from lawsuits, and the role of risk management in minimizing the number and effect of lawsuits.

The imaging professional is exposed constantly to situations that can become the subject of litigation without warning. As providers of medical imaging services, they can be required to participate in litigation. To be prepared, the imaging professional must have a basic understanding of the mechanics of a lawsuit.

THE LAWSUIT

A lawsuit is generally comprised of a pleading phase, discovery phase, and trial. During the pleading phase a complaint is lodged and an answer given. Attorneys seek the facts of the case by questioning the involved parties during the discovery phase. During the trial the case is presented to a judge or jury for a decision. (Table 1-2.)

There are time limitations in which lawsuits can be brought against a physician or other health professional. These time limits are called *statutes of limitation* and vary by jurisdiction. Restrictions are also placed on attorneys to file such lawsuits only after a reasonable inquiry has been made with regard to the facts of the claim. Settlement negotiations can and usually do occur before a lawsuit is ever filed, and they generally continue throughout the lawsuit. Most lawsuits are settled before trial.

Pleading Phase

A lawsuit is begun when a plaintiff files a complaint (also called a *claim* or a *petition,* depending on the court in which it is brought) against a defendant with the court. In a medical negligence lawsuit, this complaint may allege that the defendant has failed to provide treatment, has provided inadequate treatment, or has committed misconduct. The lawsuit alleges that the plaintiff has been injured as a result of the action or inaction of the defendant. Lawsuits may have many defendants, including doctors and individual care providers. In addition, the health care facility may be sued for the actions or lack of action of any of its employees and students. Notice of the filing of the lawsuit must be given to the defendant by very specific methods dictated by the particular court in which the lawsuit has been filed. The defendant must file a written answer to the allegations in the complaint within specific time frames set by the court in which the lawsuit has been filed.

Discovery Phase

The lawsuit then proceeds to the discovery phase. The purpose of discovery is to ascertain the truth concerning the incident. During the discovery phase, questions may be asked of any of the parties (including employees and students of a party) either in writing (interrogatories) or orally (depositions). Parties are under oath regardless of whether questions are oral or written. These interrogatory answers and statements from depositions will be used at trial if testimony contradicts or does not agree with these earlier statements.

The Trial

After the discovery phase is complete, the lawsuit advances to trial. The lawsuit may be dismissed or settled at any time before trial. Dismissal or settlement generally occurs if the discovery phase reveals facts that make the success of one party or the other unlikely at trial. Settlement negotiations often involve attorneys for the plaintiff, defendant, and defendant's insurance company, as well as the parties themselves. These negotiations can be through correspondence, telephone calls, and informal or formal meetings. Negotiators or mediators (generally very experienced attorneys or retired judges) are often used to bring objectivity to the negotiations and encourage the parties to settle the lawsuit. If a lawsuit proceeds to trial, any potentially relevant witness may be called. A student or staff medical imaging professional may be a party or a witness in a medical negligence case.

RISK MANAGEMENT

Litigation may arise from patient care in which the technologist is involved. Therefore the imaging professional must understand the importance of minimizing risk by thoroughly documenting, obtaining informed consent, maintaining patient confidentiality, practicing radiation protection, and maintaining a safe environment for patients and employees.

Risk management is the system for identifying, analyzing, and evaluating risks and selecting the most advantageous method for treating them.[15] The goal of risk management is to maintain quality patient care and conserve the facility's financial resources. An effective risk management program has three primary goals:

RISK MANAGEMENT
Risk management is the system for identifying, analyzing, and evaluating risks and selecting the most advantageous method for treating them. Its goal is to maintain quality patient care and conserve the facility's financial resources.

1. Elimination of the causes of loss experienced by the hospital and its patients, employees, and visitors
2. Lessening of the operational and financial effects of unavoidable losses
3. Covering of inevitable losses at the lowest cost

Risk management seeks to maintain quality patient care and the safety and security of the facility's patients, employees, visitors, and property. Some facilities have separate quality assurance programs focusing on quality of patient care. Others integrate risk management and quality assurance. In assessing patient care, quality assurance considers a wide range of concerns and uses hospital committees to oversee the quality of various hospital functions. These committees perform functions ranging from overseeing the quality and necessity of surgery to the determination of which doctors may practice in the hospital and what procedures they may per-

QUALITY ASSURANCE
Quality assurance is a process to assess quality of patient care that uses hospital committees to oversee the quality of various hospital functions.

BOX 1-4 COMMON RISK MANAGEMENT GUIDELINES

- Follow facility and departmental policies and procedures.
- Take a thorough, consistent, and systematic approach to informed consent and documentation.
- Strictly respect patient confidentiality.
- Practice consistent radiation protection.
- Be aware of safety issues.
- Report hazardous conditions.

IMAGING SCENARIO

A patient arrives at the imaging department for an intravenous pyelogram (IVP). The imaging technologist assigned to IVPs that day proceeds to take the patient history. During the course of the history the patient responds to a question regarding food allergies by saying she is allergic to seafood. This allergy may indicate an allergy to the iodinated contrast material used to perform an IVP. The discovery of this allergy leads the technologist to consult the radiologist, who determines that the iodinated contrast should not be used.

The discovery of this seafood allergy and the taking of appropriate action by the technologist prevented what could have been a situation likely to involve litigation. The technologist discovered this allergy because of a consistent, systematic, and thorough approach to documentation of the patient history. The advantage of the consistent, systematic, and thorough approach is that the technologist follows the same procedure with every patient, eliminating the risk of overlooking an important item of patient history.

form. Although quality assurance is an important function in patient care, for purposes of this text we will discuss risk management as including quality assurance.

Health care facilities generally employ a risk manager or a team of risk managers to maintain efficiency and quality of care. However, each student or staff imaging professional must take responsibility as a risk manager and be aware that risk is always present.

Policies and procedures are formulated in facilities and individual departments to minimize risk exposure (Box 1-4). Examples of important procedures include taking a thorough, consistent, and systematic approach to informed consent and documentation (see imaging scenario above), strictly respecting patient confidentiality, consistently practicing radiation protection, being aware of safety issues, and reporting hazardous conditions immediately. These procedures limit the litigation risks inherent in the imaging professions.

SUMMARY

Imaging professionals often must deal with dilemmas requiring ethical decision making. These dilemmas must be handled professionally. Imaging professionals rely on personal ethics derived from their value systems and professional ethics as defined in codes of ethics to make decisions regarding appropriate activities and attitudes concerning patients and other health care professionals. Their personal, cultural, and professional values also affect the ethical decision-making process. These values may conflict with each other and with those of patients and other health care providers during ethical dilemmas.

Ethical theories and models serve as tools in problem solving. The three schools of ethical thought are teleology, deontology, and virtue ethics. In addition, ethical models are employed by imaging professionals to guide patient interaction. Common models include the engineering, paternal or priestly, collegial, contractual, and covenantal models. Finally, case study analysis is aided by a decision-making framework in which the imaging professional asks questions about the context of an ethical problem and ascertains the significance to the other parties of the conflict and the values involved to determine a satisfactory outcome and avoid future ethical dilemmas.

Legal matters also may affect imaging professionals. Law has been established through common law, case law, and statutes, all of which have binding legal force. Law also may be divided into administrative, criminal, and civil law. Lawsuits involving the imaging professional are generally brought under tort law, a subdivision of civil law.

Imaging professionals are exposed constantly to situations that may result in liability for themselves, the facilities in which they work, and the physicians with whom they work. These lawsuits usually allege that harm has occurred because of negligent conduct or intentional misconduct by a health care provider. Possible roles for imaging professionals in a civil lawsuit include witness and defendant. Both roles require participation in the pleading, discovery, and trial phases of the lawsuit.

Litigation may be reduced through risk management, which seeks to improve patient care and minimize litigation risks through standardized procedures and guidelines. In addition to the established risk management team, each imaging professional must be a risk manager.

ENDNOTES

1. *Webster's new world dictionary of the American language,* ed 2, New York, 1982, Simon and Schuster.
2. Warner SB: Code of ethics: professional & legal implications, *Radiol Technol* 52(5):485, 1981.
3. American Philosophical Association: *The Delphi Report: research findings and recommendations prepared for the committee of pre-college philosophy,* ERIC Document Reproduction Service No. ED 315-423, Newark, Del., 1990.
4. Omery A: Values, moral reasoning, and ethics, *Nurs Clin North Am* 24(2):488, 1989.
5. Rokeach M: *Beliefs, attitudes, and values,* San Francisco, 1968, Jossey-Bass.
6. Fry ST: *Ethics in nursing practice: a guide to ethical decision making,* Geneva, Switzerland, 1994, International Council of Nurses.
7. Creasia J, Parker B: *Conceptual foundations of professional nursing practice,* ed 2, St Louis, 1996, Mosby.
8. Burnard P, Chapman CM: *Professional and ethical issues in nursing,* New York, 1988, John Wiley & Sons.
9. Anderson KN: *Mosby's medical, nursing, and allied health dictionary,* ed 5, St Louis, 1997, Mosby.

10. *Black's law dictionary,* ed 6, St. Paul, Minn., 1990, West.
11. *People v Rehman,* 253 C.A. 2d 119,61 Cal. Rptr. 65, 85.
12. *Smith v Weaver,* 407 N.W. 2d 174 (Neb. 1987).
13. *Korman v Mallin,* 858 P. 2d 1145 (Alaska 1993).
14. Prosser W, Wade J, Schwartz V: *Cases and materials on torts,* ed 8, Westbury, NY, 1988, Foundation Press.
15. Federation of American Health Systems: *Risk management manual,* Little Rock, Ark., 1977, Federation of American Hospitals.

REVIEW QUESTIONS

1 Biomedical ethics includes which of the following?
 a. Exact rules
 b. Feelings and beliefs of the imaging professional
 c. Legal issues and judicial decisions
 d. Guidelines from the American Medical Association
 e. All of the above

2 Consequentialism is another name for which of the following?
 a. Virtue ethics
 b. A contract
 c. Exact rules
 d. Teleology

3 Deontology emphasizes which of the following?
 a. Significance of the motives
 b. Good of the majority
 c. Emotional problem solving
 d. Practical reasoning

4 The imaging professional may encounter biomedical ethical problems because of which of the following?
 a. Value conflicts
 b. Patients' awareness or lack of awareness of rights
 c. Differing hierarchies of values
 d. All the above

5 Describe two major functions of a code of ethics.

6 The ethical model that treats the relationship between the health care provider and patient as a business agreement is the ________________ model.

7 The ____________________ model treats the provider as an omniscient or fatherlike figure.

8 The ____________________ model is based on traditional values and goals.

9 Three types of values are ______________, ______________, and ______________.

10 What four questions may help the imaging specialist solve ethical problems?
 a. ____
 b. ____
 c. ____
 d. ____

11 The origin of the current law is which of the following?
a. Common law
b. Statutes
c. Judicial decisions
d. All of the above

12 Common law is which of the following?
a. The law of common sense
b. The laws of the particular jurisdiction
c. Based on ancient usages and customs
d. The law of the common persons in England

13 An incident between a patient and an imaging technologist could involve which of the following?
a. Administrative law
b. Criminal law
c. Civil law
d. All of the above

14 Lawsuits involving the medical imaging sciences generally are brought under which kind of law?
a. Criminal law
b. Administrative law
c. Civil law, tort division
d. Common law

15 Risk management strives to do which of the following?
a. Eliminate the causes of loss in the facility
b. Lessen the effects of unavoidable losses
c. Cover inevitable costs at the lowest price
d. All of the above

16 Risk management is performed by which of the following?
a. A risk manager
b. A risk management team
c. The imaging technologist
d. All of the above

17 Risk management tools include which of the following?
a. Knowing and following policies and procedures
b. Respecting patient confidentiality
c. Practicing radiation protection
d. All of the above

18 Quality assurance uses which of the following?
a. Report cards for employees
b. Hospital committees to oversee quality issues
c. Hall monitors to watch for mistakes
d. Inspection teams to check cleaning of facility

19 **True or False** Professionalism promotes the good of the individual and depends on high ethical standards.

20 **True or False** Patients share in the responsibility for their health care.

21 **True or False** Because health care facilities have legal counsel, imaging professionals do not need to know anything about the law.
22 **True or False** Current law has been established through common law, statutes, and judicial decisions.
23 **True or False** Lawsuits involving imaging professionals are most frequently brought under criminal law.
24 **True or False** A tort action alleges harm caused by the negligent or intentional act of another.
25 **True or False** An imaging professional never has to worry about answering questions or testifying in a lawsuit.
26 **True or False** An imaging professional's role in a lawsuit may include being a witness or a defendant.
27 **True or False** Written answers to interrogatories are not important; the only information that is important is that presented at trial.
28 **True or False** Risk management is performed by the risk management department, and the imaging professional does not have to be concerned with it.
29 **True or False** The imaging professional should understand the elements of torts.
30 **True or False** Tort actions can only be brought if a patient is harmed by the intentional act of an imaging professional.
31 **True or False** An imaging professional's involvement in the discovery phase of a trial has no influence on whether the case proceeds to trial.

CRITICAL THINKING QUESTIONS & ACTIVITIES

1 Why is ethics important to the development of professional status for imaging professionals?
2 If you had to pick an ethical theory with which you felt most comfortable to aid in problem solving in imaging, which one would you choose and why?
3 To what extent should imaging professionals' religious beliefs, cultural views, values, and understanding of professional codes of ethics influence their decision making? In what way do ethical models give structure to problem-solving techniques? Give an example and justify your decision.
4 Describe the way the roles of the imaging professional and patient interact when a biomedical ethical problem develops in one of the imaging modalities. Do the roles ever conflict? Explain your reasoning.
5 Do you believe ethics is a necessary academic course for imaging professionals or is ethics common sense? Defend your answer.
6 Does imaging practice provide unique ethical dilemmas? Discuss them.

CRITICAL THINKING QUESTIONS & ACTIVITIES—cont'd

7. What is your possible involvement in each of the three phases of a lawsuit?
8. If a case proceeds to trial, in what way would your involvement in the discovery phase influence the trial?
9. Describe ways in which each imaging professional can be a risk manager.
10. What strategies do you need to learn from the next three chapters to protect yourself, your facility, and the primary care physician from liability?
11. Discuss an ethical dilemma you have personally experienced.
12. Analyze your current problem-solving skills for strengths and weaknesses.
13. Interview imaging professionals who have been in practice for 10 years or more and ask about ethical dilemmas they have observed and experienced.
14. Keep an ethical diary (individually or as a class). Include situations, questions, and personal thoughts.
15. Prepare a table listing the three schools of thought for ethical problem solving citing the precepts, similarities, and differences of each.
16. Assign teams to role play an ethical problem-solving situation in one of the imaging modalities. The ethical problem should be the same for each team, but the model and theory should vary. After the team assignments are completed, discuss application of models and theories. Cite the positive and negative aspects of each.
17. Videotape a procedure for further team development. Evaluate images, adequacy of protection, and appropriateness of positioning, and discuss patient care.

WHAT IMPACT DO ETHICAL ISSUES HAVE ON YOUR PROFESSIONAL LIFE?

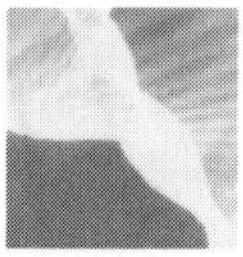

AS RADIOGRAPHERS, we do not practice our profession within a vacuum. The courses of action we choose influence patients, family members, and others in our communities. It is my belief that a sacred trust has been bestowed on us by societal norms and customs. However, this trust must be earned by each health care professional through arduous hours of study in clinical and didactic areas within a professional curriculum. It is not a given that a radiographer is empowered with trust. Just as a toddler takes somewhat precarious steps before learning to run, novice radiographers must obtain necessary self-confidence as they interact with patients in an ethical and caring manner. After repeated patient care interactions, the radiographer's sincerity should allow the patient to then open the door to trust the imaging professional. For some, this process may not be easy, whereas others may consider it second nature. Can we teach ethical behaviors to student radiographers? The cognitive information and knowledge may be presented didactically, but the student radiographer must be capable of embracing ethical behavior and placing a value on it for professional practice. Learning exercises to instill these behaviors include role playing or case study development for prescribed medicolegal issues.

We no longer have the luxury of society respecting us for wearing white coats and working in hospitals. More than appearance is required to be a professional. The demeanor in which we carry ourselves combined with our clinical expertise is often perceived favorably by patients. They want substance to back up the professional uniform. The ethical principles of beneficence, nonmaleficence, justice, and autonomy allow me to focus my attention on patients and their needs. Although we all acquire a degree of prejudice during our lives, the health care setting is not an appropriate place to exercise these maladaptive thought processes. Justice requires the radiographer to treat every patient with the highest degree of care and compassion. Today, patients are quite involved in health care decisions. Therefore autonomy or self-direction should be maintained for patients who are mentally competent. I think of beneficence as the way I may benefit my patients. I want to add to their being rather than take away from their personhood. This sounds quite esoteric, but looking within to find a personal ethical philosophy can be revealing. Nonmaleficence is intrinsic to patient care. Ob-viously, no harm should be done to patients. Some state laws now require police background checks for any individual seeking a career or employment in a patient care setting. I applaud these efforts because they may prevent harm from being done to a patient.

STEVEN D. WALTERS, MSRT(R)
DIRECTOR OF RADIOLOGY
LEE MEMORIAL HOSPITAL
Dowagiac, Michigan

CHAPTER 2

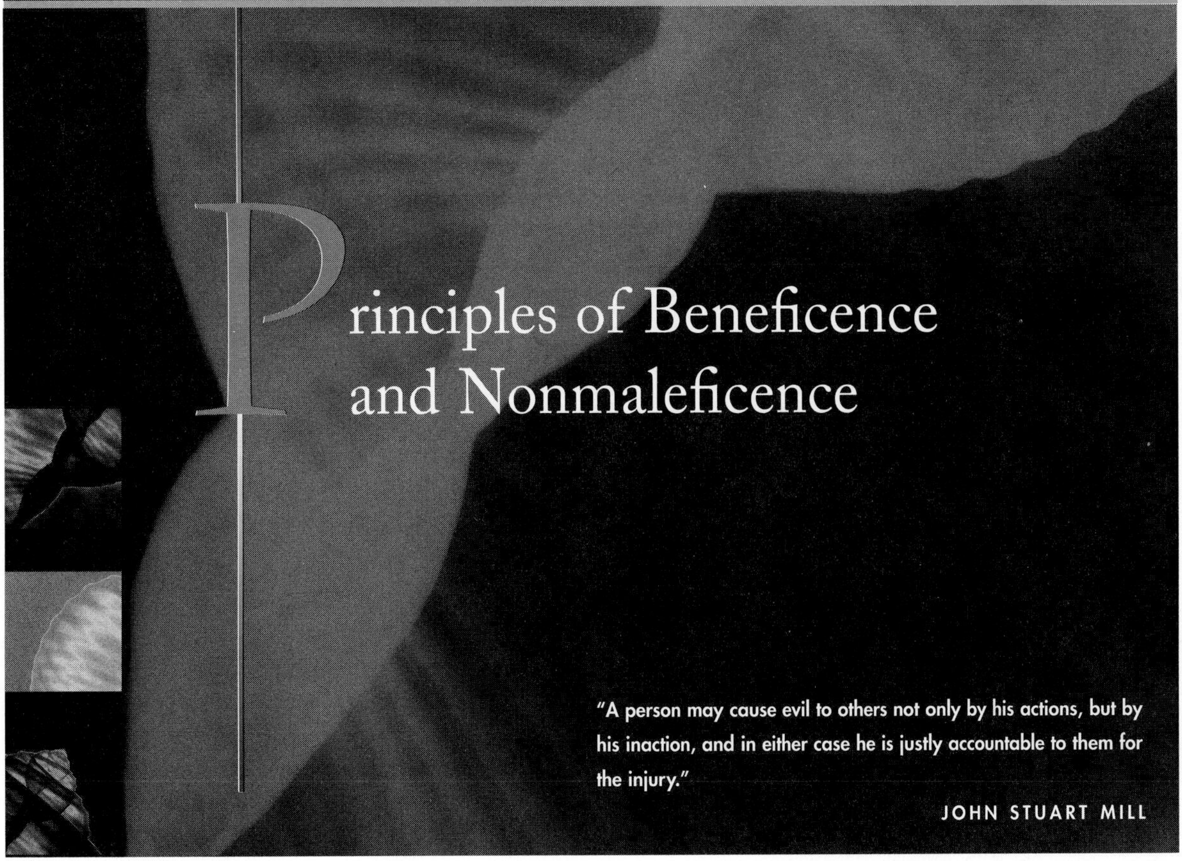

Principles of Beneficence and Nonmaleficence

"A person may cause evil to others not only by his actions, but by his inaction, and in either case he is justly accountable to them for the injury."

JOHN STUART MILL

LEARNING OBJECTIVES

- Distinguish between beneficence and nonmaleficence.
- Identify the four conditions used to assess the proportionality of good and evil in an action.
- Make appropriate decisions by applying the principles of beneficence and nonmaleficence.
- Describe the imaging professional's role in doing good and avoiding evil.
- Provide patients the necessary knowledge to ensure their participation in decision making.
- Explore and discuss the legal concept of standard of care.
- Define negligence, medical negligence, and *res ipsa loquitur.*
- Identify methods to decrease risk, including documentation, radiation protection, and safety.
- Identify and justify which information is appropriate and inappropriate for documentation.

CHAPTER OUTLINE

ETHICAL ISSUES
Proportionality
Beneficence
Nonmaleficence
Differences between Beneficence and Nonmaleficence
Justice
Contractual Agreements
Surrogate Obligations
Imaging Professional's Role
Patient's Role

LEGAL ISSUES
Standard of Care
Negligence
- Medical negligence

Methods to Decrease Risk
- Documentation (Appendix B)
  - Patient data sheet
  - Inappropriate documentation
- Incident reporting
- Documentation of the introduction of intravenous contrast material and radiopharmaceuticals
- Radiation protection
- Safety

SUMMARY

ETHICAL ISSUES

Health care decision-making processes require the consideration of all aspects of a problem. When the health care team and patient must decide whether to perform an invasive imaging procedure or drastic surgery, the team must intend good for the patient. Moreover, they must consider whether this good outweighs the risks of evil consequences.

Two integral components of decision making in medical ethics are beneficence, or the performance of good acts, and nonmaleficence, or the avoidance of evil. These two definitions may sound similar, but a closer examination reveals distinctions between the two.

This chapter explores beneficence and nonmaleficence and the ways they relate to the roles of the imaging professional and patient. It also considers justice and patient autonomy and the ways in which pursuit of those values may conflict with the ideals of beneficence and nonmaleficence.

Society expects health care professionals "to do good" and thus aid patients. This has long been an expectation of health care professionals; indeed, the Hippocratic oath begins with the exhortation to "first, do no harm."

This good encompasses proper behavior within "law, custom, relationship, and contract."[1] State and federal laws, which presumably have been based on moral and culturally virtuous processes, may give the health care professional defined guidelines within which to do good as society sees matters. For example, society perceives caring for sick people and supplying quality imaging services as inherently good. Custom further helps define good behavior based on repeated patterns within the society. Relationships between individuals, individuals and institutions, and individuals and society also contribute toward a definition of good within a society.

IMAGING SCENARIO

A male child of 4 years with Down syndrome is scheduled for a cardiac catheterization. The completed test shows a defect that will drastically limit the child's life expectancy if left untreated. The pediatric cardiologist does not recommend surgery because of the child's low intelligence quotient (IQ).

The child's parents are afraid the little boy will outlive them if he has the surgery. A vascular imaging technologist who assisted with the cardiac catheterization is horrified when she finds out the young child will not be operated on because of low IQ, inconvenience, and quality of life decisions made for the child by others. She wonders whose good the parents and doctor are considering and in what way they arrived at such a decision?

Discussion question

- In what various ways do law, custom, relationship, and contract interact in this scenario?

Additionally, the contractual process also may indicate an individual's conception of a good act.

PROPORTIONALITY

The avoidance of all evil is impossible. Because of this, society tends to value the utilitarian theory described by philosopher John Stuart Mill in which the ideal is to do the most good for the most people. However, in the achievement of good, people may be subjected to the opposite—namely, harm. For example, chemotherapy may achieve its goal of curing cancer only after causing the patient pain, nausea, and hair loss. Individuals and society therefore need to determine the amount of harm or evil that may be tolerated. To make this determination, society often applies the principle of double effect, which states that a person may perform an act that has evil effects or risk such effects as long as four conditions are met:

PRINCIPLE OF DOUBLE EFFECT
A person may perform an act that has evil effects or risk such effects as long as four certain conditions are met.

1. The action must be good or morally indifferent in itself. For example, a proposed imaging procedure must help the patient or at least not cause harm.
2. The agent must intend only the good effect and not the evil effect. That is, the imaging technologist must intend for the imaging to aid in the health care process, not injure the patient or cause pain.
3. The evil effect cannot be a means to the good effect. This condition may be complicated for the imaging technologist. The patient may believe the imaging procedure to be an evil effect; however, to gain a diagnosis, or good effect, the patient may have to undergo an unpleasant examination.
4. Proportionality must exist between good and evil effects. The good of the procedure must at least balance with the unintended pain or discomfort.

To conform to the principle of proportionality, "the action should not infringe against the good of the individual. There also has to be a proportionate good to justify the risk of an evil consequence."[1] The following questions may be used to define proportionality:

Are alternatives with less evil consequences available? May another procedure produce the same diagnosis with less pain? For example, might magnetic resonance imaging (MRI) be used instead of a myelogram?

What are the levels of good intended and evil risked? What will be gained from the procedure? For example, can the administration of a barium enema (BE) radiographic examination to a 98-year-old comatose patient with cancer be justified?

What is the probability of the good or evil intended being achieved, and what action and influence do the health care team and patient have? What gains to the patient are possible, and will the imaging specialist have to convince the patient or surrogate to have the procedure?

BENEFICENCE
Performance of good acts.

BENEFICENCE

The term *beneficence* may encompass many aspects of goodness, promoting good action and preventing evil or harm. Beneficence requires the action of an imaging professional to do good or prevent harm. For example, a patient scheduled for an invasive imaging examination may have determined that he or she does not wish to risk the possibility of the complications that may be encountered from the procedure. The imaging professional may then have to share these concerns with the radiologist and speak on behalf of the patient. A clear definition of nonmaleficence, or the avoidance of evil, may therefore aid in the critical consideration of beneficence.

NONMALEFICENCE

NONMALEFICENCE
The avoidance of evil.

Nonmaleficence, or the avoidance of evil, hinges on a system of weighting. It does not require individual action. It only requires the imaging professional to do no harm. The good desired must outweigh the risk of evil. For example, the performance of a balloon angioplasty offers the patient the great good of opening the coronary artery and enhancing the patient's quality of life. However, the health care team and patient must consider the risk of plaque dislodging within the artery and producing myocardial infarction, stroke, or death. The team weighs the possible good and evil outcomes of the procedure by assessing the physical, mental, and emotional ability of the patient to understand the risk and significance of the possible harm. If the patient is otherwise healthy, the intended good usually outweighs the unintended evil; however, if the patient already has suffered heart damage or has serious respiratory disease, the evil consequences may overshadow the intended good. The performance of good and the avoidance of evil both benefit the patient. Thus a decision must be made by weighing both good and evil.

DIFFERENCES BETWEEN BENEFICENCE AND NONMALEFICENCE

Beneficence and nonmaleficence differ in the degree of force each possesses. The stronger action of the two is nonmaleficence, or the avoidance of harm; beneficence, or the performance of good, is weaker. Although the interest of imaging professionals is in doing good, they must not cause harm while doing so. This is a vital consideration in the practice of imaging. For example, an elderly patient may have arrived in the imaging department for a dorsal spine image. The patient has a kyphosis and is crippled with degenerative arthritis and finds lying on the table intolerable. The guiding principle in this case may be to do no harm, even at the expense of the patient receiving the good of the diagnostic image. Decisions in health care should be made after consideration of both beneficence and nonmaleficence.

Although beneficence and nonmaleficence are both important considerations in patient autonomy, they differ in the way they are practiced. Beneficence is an active process, whereas nonmaleficence is passive (Table 2-1). This difference is evident in the following scenario.

JUSTICE

For imaging professionals, justice, or the principle of fairness, requires the performance of an appropriate procedure only after informed consent has been granted. Informed consent is permission, usually in writing, given by a patient agreeing to the

TABLE 2-1 DIFFERENCES BETWEEN NONMALEFICENCE AND BENEFICENCE

Nonmaleficence	Beneficence
Goal is to do no harm	Goal is to do good
Achieved through passive omission	Achieved through active process
Primary responsibility of the health care provider	Secondary in importance to nonmaleficence

IMAGING SCENARIO

A female patient is scheduled for a lumbar spine imaging series. The imaging professional in charge of the examination is interrupted and called to the emergency room to care for victims of a massive accident. Another imaging professional takes over the examination before the initial exposure is taken. When asked if everything is ready, the first technologist says "yes" and hurries to the emergency room. The second imaging technologist surveys the patient, who is covered with a sheet, introduces himself, and then performs the lumbar spine series. The processed images reveal that the woman is in her first trimester of pregnancy. Obviously, an injustice has been done, and a lawsuit may possibly result. Was the injustice active—did the first or second imaging professional deliberately not shield the patient and ask about possible pregnancy? Conversely, was the injustice an unintentional error of omission resulting from the confusion caused by the first technologist leaving to attend to accident victims in the emergency room? If the case is decided in court, the ruling may be affected by whether the injustice was a result of active intent or passive omission. The obligation not to harm is the strongest motivator in medicine, but the avoidance of evil also is essential.

performance of a procedure. (Issues of informed consent are developed more fully in Chapter 3.) Conflicts among beneficence, nonmaleficence, and autonomy (the state of independent self-government) may arise during consideration of principles of justice. The general belief in the right to health care brings beneficence and nonmaleficence into conflict with autonomy and justice. Although most people believe that the good of health care should be available to all, health care resources are limited and hard decisions must be made about their allocation. Limited resources reduce the overall quality of care and may lead to less avoidance of evil. When quality of health care is reduced, the patient's autonomy suffers from loss of freedom of choices. When choices are limited, the obligations of the patient and health care giver may conflict with resources and justice for the patient (Figure 2-1).

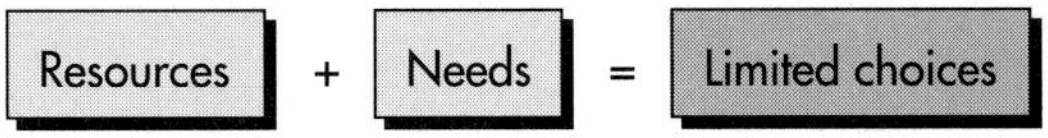

FIGURE 2-1
The needs of patients and care providers can conflict because of limited resources, making ethical decisions part of a professional's daily tasks.

The performance of good and the avoidance of evil often come into conflict when medical indication principles or the proportionality of consequences are judged by the health care provider. The medical indication principle states that, "granted informed consent, the physician should do what is medically indicated such that, from a medical point of view, more good than evil will result."[1]

The conflict between beneficence and nonmaleficence on the one hand and informed consent and patient autonomy on the other may be explored further by asking how, if the health care professional cannot make quality-of-life decisions concerning patients but must make recommendations concerning good and evil, can decision making lead to patient autonomy? For example, an imaging professional may be asked to give an imaging examination to a neonate in intensive care. The infant has the majority of its organs outside of the abdomen, including a massive spina bifida. The imaging professional wonders why the infant's life is being maintained by artificial methods. However, this question is an issue for the family. It is not the imaging professional's responsibility to make quality-of-life decisions for others.

CONTRACTUAL AGREEMENTS

Verbal and written contractual agreements help provide for patient autonomy. Patients requiring imaging services enter into contractual agreements when they agree to enter a hospital and undergo a series of diagnostic imaging studies. Usually such contracts take the form of blanket statements of informed consent. They are general agreements; other processes of informed consent may be required as specific procedures are scheduled. The processes of informed consent and the procedures employed in providing it are discussed at length in Chapter 3.

SURROGATE OBLIGATIONS

Another area of conflict is within surrogate obligations. The interactions among patient autonomy, beneficence, and nonmaleficence become even more complex in these situations. If the patient is incompetent, either the best interests of the patient or the rational choice principle should be used. The rational choice principle "commands that the surrogate choose what the patient would have chosen when competent and after having considered all available relevant information and the interests of the relevant others."[1] In determining the best interests of the patient, the proportionality between good and evil may be different for patient and surrogate; this may interfere with patient autonomy. In this situation the surrogate must include the patient's and perhaps significant others' attitudes regarding good and evil consequences.

IMAGING PROFESSIONAL'S ROLE

The imaging professional must be aware of the obligations to do good and avoid harm. Every imaging procedure has the potential to harm the patient; invasive procedures, radiation, and equipment malfunction all pose dangers to the patient. Maintaining a high quality of patient care and technologic skills helps ensure that procedures achieve good for the patient, and practicing protective measures aids in the avoidance of harm (Figure 2-2). Each imaging professional must be responsible for daily contact with patients receiving diagnostic health care procedures.

PATIENT'S ROLE

Patients participate in protecting their own good and avoiding their own harm by gathering information about the imaging procedure they will be undergoing. If the patient is unable to understand this information, a surrogate should be appointed to guarantee that appropriate informed consent is given, which will lead to the avoidance of harm and the doing of good. If the patient is in doubt, a second opinion should be sought.

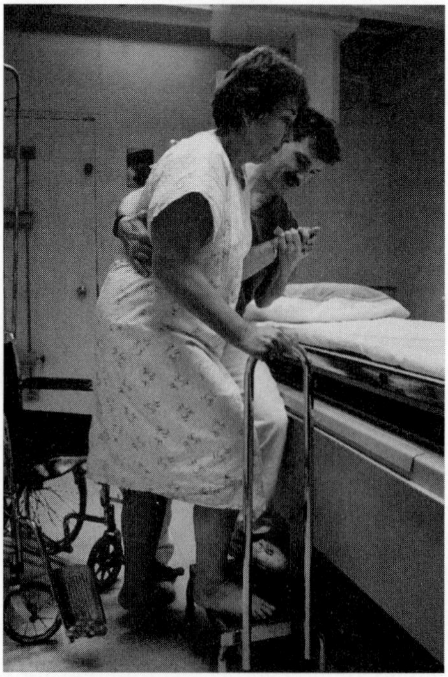

FIGURE 2-2

Safe transport of patients to, from, and within the imaging department is one way of showing both beneficence and nonmaleficence.

LEGAL ISSUES

The ethical concepts of beneficence and nonmaleficence may not generally be thought to be connected with legal theories involving health care. However, these concepts—the doing of good and avoidance of harm—may be seen to be incorporated into the duty of a health professional to do no harm and provide reasonable care to the patient. This section explores the legal concept of standard of care. The reasonable care that is expected is defined and the negative results when less than reasonable care is provided are discussed.

In addition, this section provides methods to ensure reasonable patient care is provided and litigation risk is decreased. Included in these methods are documentation, radiation protection, and safety issues.

STANDARD OF CARE

The law provides many parameters for the delivery of imaging services. These parameters have evolved from various statutes (laws written and enacted by state or federal legislatures) and court decisions. The most basic legal parameter in health care is the standard of care, which encompasses the obligation of health care professionals to do no harm and their duty to provide reasonable patient care. Standards of care are established by each profession to define the parameters within which that profession is obligated to practice. They are not limited to the imaging services but exist for all other health care providers in the facility, the physicians, and the facility itself.

STANDARD OF CARE
The degree of skill or care practiced by a reasonable professional practicing in the same field.

The legal standard is the degree of skill or care employed by a reasonable professional practicing in the same field.[2] Lack of training or experience is not an excuse for the failure of a health care professional to perform a duty to the patient adequately. For example, imaging professionals working as nuclear medicine technologists are held to the same standard of care as trained and certified nuclear medicine technologists. If the appropriate standard of care is violated, liability may be imposed on both health care professionals and medical facilities.

Scope of practice, educational requirements, and curricula developed for the medical imaging sciences all help to establish the standard of care to which imaging professionals must hold themselves. The scope of practice for health care specialists is set forth by that discipline's national professional organization. It is generally a series of guidelines to determine what health care specialists should or should not do under certain circumstances.[3] Standards for accreditation for educational programs in radiologic sciences as defined by the Joint Review Committee on Education in Radiologic Technology (effective January 1997)[4] or other regional accreditation agencies with similar standards must be met for graduates to be recognized by the American Registry of Radiologic Technologists (ARRT). ARRT recognition is generally a requirement for reimbursement by Medicare, Medicaid, and many private insurers.

Imaging professionals must maintain knowledge of the current standard of care. This is particularly important the longer an imaging professional is out of the educational program. The radiologic sciences are changing rapidly. Those practicing in these fields have an obligation to update their knowledge and remain current as these changes occur. Attending appropriate continuing education programs and reading professional publications are both methods that can be used to keep abreast of the current standard of care. Every patient receiving imaging services is entitled to expect the same level of care as the standard of care recognized by the law.

NEGLIGENCE

NEGLIGENCE
An unintentional tort involving duty, breach of duty, injury, and causation.

REASONABLE CARE
The degree of care a reasonable person, similarly situated, would use.

Negligence is an unintentional tort resulting from actions not intended to do harm. It occurs in situations in which a duty to use reasonable care is owed to another and an injury results from a failure to use reasonable care. Reasonable care is the degree of care a reasonable person, similarly situated, would use. Reasonable care may be determined by the applicable standard of care, by statute, or by previous judicial decisions, called precedents.[5] If a duty is not performed with reasonable care, liability may be imposed.

Negligence requires a duty, a breach of that duty, injury, and causation. For example, if a driver falls asleep at the wheel, crosses the center line, strikes another car, and injures its driver, the driver has been negligent. Statutes and precedents have established that all drivers have a duty to share the road reasonably with other drivers. The driver who fell asleep and crossed the center line was not acting reasonably. The other driver's injuries were a direct result of the first driver's failure to act reasonably. The driver who crossed the center line was negligent and is liable for damages.

Medical Negligence

A special relationship exists between health care providers and patients. This special relationship entails a duty on the part of the health care professional to provide patients with reasonable care. Whether reasonable care is provided is determined by the standard of care for whatever is done to the patient. A health care provider's failure to follow the appropriate standard of care is therefore a special type of negligence called *medical negligence.* This type of negligence is sometimes referred to under the general term of *medical malpractice.*

MEDICAL NEGLIGENCE
A breach of the health care provider's duty to follow the applicable standard of care that results in harm to the patient.

A medical imaging professional owes a duty to the patient to ensure that procedures are performed according to the applicable standard of care. That standard of care requires the imaging professional to follow accepted guidelines for that procedure. A deviation from those guidelines that causes harm to a patient may form the basis for a judgment of liability. Although variations exist between jurisdictions, generally a plaintiff must provide evidence establishing an applicable standard of care, demonstrate that the standard has been violated, and prove a causal relationship between the violation and the alleged harm.[6]

The applicable standard of care is generally established through the testimony of a medical expert practicing in the same field as the defendant. A plaintiff must offer proof that the defendant breached this legally required standard of care and thus was negligent. Expert testimony is needed to establish both the proper standard of care and a failure by the defendant to conform to that standard.[7] An exception to the requirement of an expert witness exists in situations where a layperson could understand the negligence without the assistance of experts.[8]

If a lawsuit proceeds to trial, the imaging professional may have an opportunity to provide his or her personal recollections of the events. However, written documentation is extremely important; attorneys, judges, and juries may indeed take the position that if an event was not documented, it did not happen. As stated earlier, expert medical testimony often is required in medical negligence suits to help the jury determine the standard of care to be applied and whether the actions of the individual violated that standard.

Medical imaging professionals have an obligation to perform examinations in a manner consistent with policies and procedures, never vary from accepted standards of care, and provide appropriate documentation. These and other methods to decrease risk are discussed thoroughly later in this chapter.

The legal doctrine of *res ipsa loquitur* (Latin for "the thing speaks for itself") may have a significant impact on medical malpractice cases. It is applicable in situations in which a particular injury would not have occurred in the absence of negligence and is often used as a basis for lawsuits arising from sponges or instruments being left in a patient after surgery.

RES IPSA LOQUITUR
Latin term meaning "the thing speaks for itself." It is a legal concept invoked in situations in which a particular injury could not have occurred in the absence of negligence.

When *res ipsa loquitur* is claimed as the basis for a lawsuit, all parties involved in the procedure are defendants because obviously at least one of them was negligent. They all must therefore try to prove that they were not negligent. Many examples exist in the medical imaging practice to which the doctrine may apply. For example, a confused elderly patient left alone on a cart in the hall after a procedure may fall and suffer a broken hip. The fall and injury would not have happened if the patient had not been left alone in the hall without being appropriately restrained. Therefore all health care professionals who worked with the patient, including the imaging specialists, may be called on to prove absence of negligence. Expert testimony may be used to prove the standard of care was violated. However, if a clear breach of duty is evident to a layperson after the presentation of the facts of the case, expert testimony may not even be needed.

METHODS TO DECREASE RISK

Documentation (Appendix B)

The type of information to be documented and incorporated into the patient record is a crucial consideration for medical professionals, but one that has not been made entirely clear. From a legal perspective, certain information is mandated by statutes, regulations, and institutional requirements. The Code of Ethics adopted by the ASRT and ARRT requires the radiologic technologist to act as an agent through observation and communication to obtain pertinent information to aid in the diagnosis and treatment of the patient.[9] Joint Commission on Accreditation of Health Care Organizations (JCAHO) regulations require that pertinent patient histories be taken on all procedures performed in the medical imaging sciences. Departmental policies generally mandate that this information be recorded on every patient record. (See Appendix B for sample patient data sheet and incident report.)

Other than the basic information mandated by statutory, regulatory, ethical, and institutional requirements, no steadfast rules govern the documentation of additional information in the medical imaging sciences. However, an examination of the purposes of documentation may help the imaging professional make decisions regarding the inclusion of additional patient information.

Quality patient care in the imaging sciences, particularly accurate diagnosis in diagnostic procedures and correct application of therapeutic radiography, depends largely on the interpreting physician receiving pertinent information about the patient. The imaging professional must communicate with the patient, observe the patient, and interpret responses and observations. This process helps the professional formulate the patient's pertinent history. Often judgments are made regarding examinations to be performed and specific positioning to be used based on the patient's history. Moreover, the interpreting physician may not be able to analyze images correctly and make accurate diagnoses without the information contained in an accurate and pertinent patient history.

However, even the information necessary to ensure the correct procedure is performed properly and interpreted accurately may not be adequate to protect health

IMAGING SCENARIO

An imaging professional and radiologist perform a venogram on a patient with diabetes. Almost 2 years later a lawsuit is filed alleging that the venogram was performed improperly. The specific allegation is that the intravenous administration of some of the contrast medium failed, causing the fluid to infiltrate the soft tissues of the foot. The suit further alleges that the infiltration caused a cellulitis to develop, and the cellulitis has resulted in continuing pain and the patient's inability to bear weight on the extremity. The imaging professional is told that she is likely to be deposed and receives from the hospital's legal department a set of questions to be answered under oath:

Discussion questions

- How much do you remember about the procedure?
- Did you document the procedure?
- How thorough was your documentation?
- Did it include documentation of the number of injections and injection sites?
- Did you document any patient complaints at the time?
- Did you document any report of patient status at the conclusion of the examination indicating the patient had no complaints?
- Did you document your observations on a form that became a permanent record along with the patient's images?
- Did the images you took include the injection sites and the area of diagnostic interest?
- Is documentation available to prove that the risks of the procedure were explained to the patient and the patient understood?

care professionals and the medical facility. Thus imaging professionals must consider ways to obtain enough information to minimize the litigation risks.

As the previous scenario indicates, remembering all the details of the particular procedure performed is extremely difficult. Written and radiographic documentation is a great aid in the defense of an unfounded medical negligence case. Imaging professionals have the opportunity and obligation to document thoroughly and thus avoid or minimize the effects of unfounded medical negligence claims (Box 2-1).

Patient Data Sheet

A uniform patient data sheet or computerized form must be developed for use in each facility (Box 2-2). Input from the department administrator, risk manager, physicians, and legal counsel in the drafting of this form is advisable.

BOX 2-1 DOCUMENTATION BASICS

Never alter or falsify a record. You will lose all credibility if alteration or falsification of records is discovered.

If you make an error, draw a line through it and write "error." Never use correction fluid or put a sticker over an error. Others must be able to see clearly the information you have changed in order for you to maintain credibility.

Know and adhere to your department's policies and guidelines. They help define expectations of reasonable care in your facility and may be evaluated in a lawsuit to determine whether your actions complied.

Document clearly and in chronologic order. If comments are necessary, make them in chronologic order. Do not leave blanks to fill in later. Blank spaces give the impression that the documentation was altered or sanitized.

Record accurate and complete information. If a problem occurred, document the action taken in response. For example, if the patient has a contrast reaction, note it and the resulting treatment.

Do not document irrelevant details.

Provide objective, factual information. Avoid conclusory terms such as well, good, fine, and normal.

Sign your legal name and title and always make your documentation legible. Illegible writing can only hurt you if litigation results.

Keep records in a safe place and respect confidentiality. The maintenance of patient confidentiality is a duty of each member of the health care team. Documentation in a medical imaging department carries the same obligation of patient confidentiality as does the information in the patient's chart.

Use incident reports to report unusual circumstances. Do not refer to incident reports in routine documentation. The incident report is for use in quality assurance and risk management to improve patient care. Acknowledgment of it in routine documentation may change it from a patient care improvement tool to a discoverable document in a lawsuit.

Modified from McMullen P, Philipsen N: Charting basics 101, *Nurs Connect* 6(3):62, 1993.

BOX 2-2 ITEMS TO BE INCLUDED IN THE PATIENT DATA SHEET

Basic patient identification information
Pertinent patient history
Answers to questions regarding pregnancy and last menstrual period
Signature line
Time of patient arrival and departure
Name of technologist performing examination
Comment section

Generally the form should include basic patient identification information, including answers to questions used to assess for pregnancy, and pertinent patient history. A signature line for the patient and a line to note the time the patient arrived and departed from the medical imaging department also may be included. In addition, the form may indicate the imaging technologist who performed the examination and provide space for additional comments. This comment section should be used to note and explain any variance from written procedure such as the patient's refusal to cooperate during part or all of the examination. If data is collected in a computer, a comment section should be available on the computerized form or an alternative method should be available to document any variance from standard procedure. If computerized patient data documentation is used, an alternate system must be in place for the inevitable "computer-down" situations. The patient data sheet should be part of the permanent patient record.

Inappropriate Documentation

Because proper documentation is so crucial, the imaging technologist also must understand what type of information is inappropriate for documentation and the reason for this determination. Because medical records are business documents, they must reflect only factual information regarding patients and their care and treatment. Documenting personal opinions or derogatory statements regarding the patient is inappropriate and may result in liability for the imaging professional, medical facility, or both.

Incident Reporting

The incident report is a valuable risk management tool. Health care facilities require incident reports on occurrences that have resulted or may result in hospital liability or patient dissatisfaction. Examples include sudden deaths; falls; drug, contrast, and radiopharmaceutical errors and reactions; injuries caused by faulty equipment; injuries to employees or visitors; threats of legal action; and unexplained requests from attorneys for medical records. Generally, department heads and supervisors are responsible for filing incident reports, but imaging professionals should know the procedures in their facilities before the need arises.

Incident reports are generally directed to the risk manager, who investigates as necessary. The risk manager also informs appropriate administrative and medical staff, and, if necessary, the facility's insurer. The incident report is a valuable tool because it allows compilation of data to identify problem areas and thus prevent errors and injuries.

Incident reporting should not be done on the patient data sheet. The facility's risk management department has set up procedures to report incidents; these procedures should be followed. The reasons for this are twofold:

1. Risk management has put specific incident reporting procedures in place because the incident report is a valuable tool for assessing risk and tracking problems in a facility. The ultimate goal of such reports is to improve patient care.
2. From a legal perspective the patient chart, including all imaging department documentation, is discoverable in a lawsuit. Incident reports generally fall into a different category and may not be as easily discoverable. However, acknowledgment of an incident report in routine documentation may make it more easily discoverable.

Documentation of the Introduction of Intravenous Contrast Material and Radiopharmaceuticals

Any procedure performed in an imaging department that involves the intravenous (IV) administration of contrast material carries with it the risk of allergic reaction. Although these reactions may range from mild, such as an itchy nose, to severe responses, such as anaphylactic shock, the risk is great enough to mandate extensive documentation.

Procedures involving the introduction of contrast material or radiopharmaceuticals present special documentation needs. Forms for documenting the type of material administered during the examination and other important information are very useful. A standardized form with spaces for each piece of information makes the regular recording of this information much more likely (Box 2-3). However, a form is useful only if it is properly and consistently used. Imaging professionals performing risky procedures have a responsibility to ensure such proper and consistent documentation.

A form for documenting procedures involving injection of contrast medium or radiopharmaceuticals should include a place for allergies to be noted. For risk management purposes a notation should always be entered in that space, such as "no known allergies" (NKA) if the patient denies allergies. Strict adherence to this requirement ensures that the question is asked and answered every time IV contrast material is administered. The form also should include a space for recording that informed consent was obtained and the proper documentation is in the patient chart.

The form also should include space for documentation concerning basic information about the material used, including identification, amount used, time administered, path of administration (oral, IV, through catheter, rectal), name of person administering the material, and injection site or sites.

Documentation of the injection site is important for several reasons. The delivery of quality patient care, especially continuity of care, requires this documentation because of the possibility of problems developing with the injection site. Risk management concerns require the information because infiltration of contrast material

BOX 2-3 ITEMS TO BE INCLUDED IN THE INTRODUCTION OF CONTRAST MATERIAL AND RADIOPHARMACEUTICALS DATA SHEET

Documentation of the obtaining of informed consent
Allergies
Material used
Amount (volume and radioactivity if using radiopharmaceutical)
Time of administration
Path of administration (oral, IV, through catheter, rectal)
Injection sites
Name of person administering material
Reaction
Time of reaction
Symptoms of reaction
Treatment of reaction
Physician treating
Time and condition on leaving department

may raise possible litigation issues. For example, documentation of the number and location of injection sites used in venograms is extremely important. Questions on the form that prompt entering required information and spaces for responses are helpful in ensuring adequate documentation.

Space should be provided to note any reaction the patient exhibits to the contrast material. This documentation should include all reactions: nose itching requiring no treatment, hives requiring treatment with diphenhydramine (Benadryl), or full-blown anaphylactic shock reactions. Documentation of reactions should be chronologic and include the symptoms observed, actions taken in response to the reaction, and detailed descriptions of treatments initiated. The condition of the patient on leaving the radiology department and the transferring of care to other health care providers such as the nursing floor or emergency department also should be documented.

As with pharmaceuticals given on the nursing floor, pharmaceuticals given in an imaging department also should be charted. Each facility should have a facility-wide system of charting in place. All individuals authorized to record information on patient charts (including imaging professionals) should be educated regarding the charting style, including accepted abbreviations. This will ensure that charting is performed uniformly by all health care providers.

Radiation Protection

The National Council on Radiation Protection and Measurements (NCRP) establishes policies and procedures regarding radiation exposure based on the phrase "as low as reasonably achievable" or ALARA. The primary goal of utilizing this concept is to keep radiation exposure of the individual well below a level at which adverse effects are likely to be observed during the individual's lifetime. Anytime physicians order a radiographic procedure, they must weigh the benefits to be obtained against the risk of exposure.[10]

Because radiation exposure is a risk, an important task for imaging professionals is the use of proper radiation protection to provide quality patient care and reduce litigation risk. Radiation protection education is essential in keeping exposures to patients ALARA[10]:

> Methods utilized in radiation protection are use of proper exposure factors, filtration, collimation, and shielding devices. Other methods which can be employed to reduce the number of repeat exposures include restraining devices, technique charts, and a quality control program which ensures proper equipment performance. Repeat film analyses and clear policies concerning pregnant patients are also essential to keep radiation exposure as low as reasonably achievable.

Instruction in radiation protection is part of the curricula of accredited educational facilities and is documented in student records. Additionally, many states and medical facilities require continuing education in radiation protection on an established schedule.

Preventive maintenance and calibration performed routinely on equipment ensures that the radiation dose emitted is accurate and appropriate. Additionally, equipment inspection is performed periodically by state and federal agencies to ensure that proper maintenance and calibration have been performed on each piece of equipment and the equipment meets acceptable standards. Records of all preventive maintenance, calibration, and government inspections should be kept in the department.

Quality control and assurance programs are performed in the imaging department to ensure that patients do not receive unnecessary radiation. These programs include repeated examination analysis, tracking of results, and measures to correct noticed problems. These programs also ensure processing equipment is performing correctly and consistently.

Consistently following policies and procedures for shielding and collimation also help protect patients against unnecessary radiation. Pregnancy poses the greatest risks in this area. For this reason, an imaging professional should always ask a female patient whether she may be pregnant and question her about the date of her last menstrual period.

If a pregnant patient must be radiographed, informed consent should be obtained and additional shielding should always be used. The informed consent procedure must include an explanation by a physician of the risks involved in exposing the fetus to ionizing radiation. Documentation of this consent must be made. (For further information about obtaining informed consent, see Chapter 3.)

Safety

Safety is an important concern in any health care facility, both in the provision of quality patient care and the reduction of litigation risks. Larger facilities generally have comprehensive safety programs that include written policies and procedures regarding handling of hazardous materials, fire and electricity safety, emergency codes, back safety, patient transport and lifting techniques, infection control, occurrence reporting, and loss prevention. Most facilities use risk management guidelines as they develop these policies and procedures. JCAHO guidelines exist for safety programs, and institutional policies and procedures generally follow these guidelines.

IMAGING SCENARIO

A patient comes to the medical imaging department for a chest x-ray for suspected pneumonia. The routine questions regarding pregnancy are asked, and the patient states she is sure she is not pregnant but does not remember the date of her last menstrual period. On the patient data form, she answers "no" to the pregnancy question but leaves the last menstrual period space blank. She signs the signature line. She receives posteroanterior (PA) and lateral chest x-rays. Later she finds out she was approximately 4 weeks pregnant when she was radiographed. Her obstetrician calls the radiologist, concerned that the woman has been radiographed and worried about the possible harm caused to the fetus. The radiologist requests that the imaging technologist pull the films. The films demonstrate the collimation line, which shows the beam was collimated to approximately ½ inch within all edges of the film. The documentation reflects what was stated regarding the pregnancy question.

Discussion questions

- Is the radiation dose to the fetus likely to be significant? Why or why not?
- Is the technologist or facility liable for negligently exposing a fetus to ionizing radiation?
- What else could have been done to protect the fetus?
- Would the same measures have limited the risk of litigation?

IMAGING SCENARIO

A patient falls on an uneven floor between the emergency and sonography departments. The sonographer tells the patient, "We keep waiting for them to fix that spot. Several other people have fallen, and we keep telling them to fix it." The sonographer then takes the patient to the ultrasound room, performs the study, and returns the patient to the emergency department without relating the incident to anyone or filling out an incident report. The patient had complained only of a little swelling in her ankle.

Discussion questions

- Was the standard of care regarding incident reports followed?
- Were other standards not met?
- Did the statement by the sonographer have any impact on any liability issues?

NOTE: Any statement made regarding previous incidents resulting from the same hazard has a legal impact because such a statement establishes that the facility knew about the hazard and therefore breached its duty by failing to warn of the hazard or remedy it. If the patient was indeed injured in the fall, the facility would be liable for negligence. In addition, the facility would be liable for failing to follow policies and procedures for incident reporting and safety and for violating those standards of care.

Although smaller facilities may have fewer staff members to educate about safety issues, the same safety standards must be met as those expected of larger facilities. Imaging professionals should know their facility's programs and be familiar with policies and procedures. If a safety issue arises while a patient is in the imaging department, the imaging professional is responsible for knowing the correct action to take. The department should keep records of attendance at safety instruction and in-service meetings.

If imaging professionals do not know whether their facilities offer safety programs, they should find out by asking supervisors until they get an appropriate answer. If no safety program exists, JCAHO guidelines EC1, 1.1-1.9 and EC2, 2.1-2.14 are excellent starting points.[11]

SUMMARY

The values of beneficence and nonmaleficence have been respected since the times of the earliest health care providers who tried to provide a good by aiding the sick and injured. They provide a system of checks and balances for providers and patients to aid in decision-making processes concerning medical care. To facilitate this decision-making process, the principle of double effect helps weigh the proportionality between good and evil consequences. Although beneficence and nonmaleficence are both necessary to patient autonomy, some differences exist between them. Benefience is active, whereas nonmaleficence is passive; further differences are evident in the importance of the ways they are practiced.

Conflict may arise between beneficence and nonmaleficence, and this often affects patient autonomy. Conflicts may arise when good intentions have negative consequences. They also may result from friction between the notion that all people deserve good health care and the reality of limited resources, power struggles, quality-of-life decisions, and surrogate obligations.

The imaging professional and patient are both responsible for encouraging good and avoiding harm in the imaging process. Continuing education enhances the imaging professional's skills, and obtaining information concerning the procedure aids the patient in appropriate decision making.

In any pluralistic society, the many interpretations of beneficence and nonmaleficence ensure that patient autonomy remains a source and cause of conflicts. These conflicts must be addressed to provide society with appropriate health care.

The ethical concepts of beneficence and nonmaleficence, which are integrated into the legal standard of care for health care professionals, define the duty to do no harm and provide reasonable medical care. The legal standard of care is the degree of skill or care practiced by a reasonable professional practicing in the same field. The standard of care for imaging professionals is established through scope of practice, educational requirements, and curricula developed for imaging professionals. It is an important consideration if negligence is alleged.

Negligence is an unintentional tort resulting from actions not intended to cause harm. For negligence to be proved, a duty to use reasonable care must exist, this duty must be breached, and harm must result from this breach. The existence of a duty and the determination of reasonable care may be established by statutes, previous judicial decisions, or appropriate standards of care.

Health care providers have a special relationship with patients that involves a duty to follow the appropriate standard of care. If that standard is not followed, liability may ensue for the health care provider and medical facility. This is called *medical negligence* or *medical malpractice.* To establish medical negligence, a plaintiff must provide evidence of an applicable standard of care, demonstrate the standard has been violated, show that an injury occurred, and prove the injury was caused by the violation of the standard of care.

Methods to ensure quality patient care and decrease risks include thorough and consistent documentation, radiation protection, and dedication to safety. Documentation forms are useful tools in ensuring consistent documentation; examples of information to be included on these forms have been provided in this chapter.

The principles of beneficence and nonmaleficence also have an impact on patient consent, informed consent, advance directives, and surrogate decision makers. Legal issues concerning consent and informed consent are discussed in Chapter 3 in the context of patient autonomy. Legal issues regarding advance directives and surrogate decision makers are addressed in Chapter 5 in the context of choices about death and dying.

ENDNOTES

1. Garrett TA, Baillie HW, Garrett RM: *Healthcare ethics, principles and problems,* ed 2, Englewood Cliffs, NJ, 1993, Prentice Hall, p 57.
2. *Bruni v. Tatsumi,* 346 N.E. 2d 673 (Ohio 1976).
3. American Society of Radiologic Technologists: *The scopes of practice for health care professionals in the radiologic sciences,* Albuquerque, NM, 1996, Author.
4. The Joint Review Committee on Education in Radiologic Technology: *Standards for an accredited educational program in radiologic sciences,* Chicago, 1996, Author.
5. Prosser W, Wade J, Schwartz V: *Cases and materials on torts,* ed 8, Westbury, NY, 1988, Foundation Press.
6. *Kennis v. Mercy Hospital Medical Center,* 491 N.W. 2d 161 (Iowa 1992).
7. Farrow B et al: *Health law,* St. Paul, Minn., 1995, West.
8. *Bauer v. Friedland,* 394 N.W. 2d 549 (Minn. App. 1986).
9. American Society of Radiologic Technologists, American Registry of Radiologic Technologists: *Code of ethics,* Mendota Heights, Minn., 1994, Author.
10. Gurley LT, Callaway WJ: *Introduction to radiologic technology,* ed 4, St Louis, 1996, Mosby.
11. Joint Commission on Accreditation of Health Care Organizations, *Accreditation manual,* Chicago, 1994, Author.

REVIEW QUESTIONS

1 Beneficence involves which of the following?
- a. Active participation of the imaging professional
- b. Doing good
- c. Preventing harm
- d. All of the above

2 Nonmaleficence occurs when which of the following takes place?
- a. Good is done.
- b. Evil is avoided.
- c. Evil is done.
- d. Good is avoided.

3 Which of the following is a contractual agreement?
- a. Demonstration of a procedure
- b. Good intentions
- c. Informed consent processes
- d. None of the above

4 The strongest action is ________________, or the avoidance of harm; ________________ is weaker and concerns the doing of good.

5 Which four conditions are used in the principle of double effect to assess the proportionality of good and evil in an action?
- a.
- b.
- c.
- d.

6 **True or False** Taking part in continuing education and performing risk management procedures help ensure quality imaging procedures for the patient.

7 Gathering information about imaging procedures is a method of participation for ________________ in their health care.

8 Conflicts arise between ________________ and ________________ and may affect patient autonomy.

9 Explain why beneficence and nonmaleficence are important to the imaging professional. Explain their differences.

10 Give an example of an act of beneficence and an act of nonmaleficence in imaging services.

11 Which is more important: the doing of good or the avoidance of harm? In what way did you arrive at that conclusion?

12 In what way does the patient exercise personal responsibility over the proportionality of beneficence and nonmaleficence involved in the imaging procedure?

13 What is the standard of care for imaging professionals?

14 Through what mechanisms is the standard of care for imaging professionals established?

15 In a lawsuit, how are decisions regarding the appropriate standard of care and violations of those standards made?
16 Can a mistake that harms a patient create liability for negligence?
17 What four elements must exist for negligence to be proved?
18 What elements must exist for medical negligence to be proved?
19 Does the special relationship between health care providers and patients eliminate the need for a plaintiff to prove that a duty of care exists?
20 What are the purposes of documentation?
21 How can documentation decrease litigation risks?
22 What other methods to decrease risk are discussed in this chapter?
23 **True or False** Quality-of-life determinations, patient autonomy, and justice in health care delivery all require decisions involving beneficence and nonmaleficence.
24 **True or False** The imaging professional and patient are not both responsible for health care decision making.

CRITICAL THINKING QUESTIONS & ACTIVITIES

1. Cite two or three routinely performed imaging procedures that involve the weighing of good and evil. Why do these procedures require this consideration? Ask other imaging professionals whether they agree.
2. Create a table of specific imaging procedures (e.g., BEs, IPUs) that have good and evil consequences. List these goods and evils and determine situations in which one outweighs the other. Discuss this system with your classmates.
3. Discuss the active and passive omission that occurred in the imaging scenario concerning the pregnant patient. Who bears the fault in this situation? Where would you place the blame? Discuss this scenario with your imaging manager.
4. Consider an imaging situation in which ethical principles seem to conflict with one another. How would you determine the correct action? To initiate this activity, an individual should present an imaging situation offering possible good and bad consequences for the patient to the group. Each individual should then list the good and bad consequences. After all the individual lists are completed, the participants should read their lists aloud; a facilitator may record each good or bad consequence. The goods and bads should then be weighed, and a discussion of proportionality should follow. Do the goods outweigh the bads or vice versa? This exercise may help the imaging professional develop a method of decision making concerning ethical dilemmas.

CRITICAL THINKING QUESTIONS & ACTIVITIES—cont'd

5 List several factors involved in determining the imaging professional's obligation to the patient. Compare with classmates' lists.

6 Discuss ways in which you can limit the chance of making mistakes that may cause liability for medical negligence.

7 Discuss the venogram legal scenario. Does the documentation form in your department cover these issues?

8 Discuss the different outcomes in the pregnancy legal scenario if the collimation lines were not visible on the film.

9 Discuss whether you are informed about safety issues. If a fire were to break out in your department and you had a patient on the table and several waiting, what should you do? What if the fire is in another area of the hospital? What do you do if a patient slips and falls while in your care? What should you do if you notice a leaking ceiling while on your way out of the hospital?

ETHICAL AND LEGAL CONSIDERATIONS IN RADIATION THERAPY

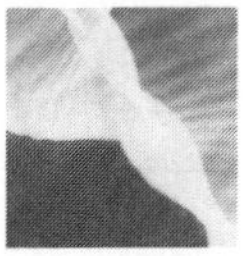

RADIATION ONCOLOGY IS BOTH AN ART AND SCIENCE, designed to deliver a prescribed dose of ionizing radiation aimed at curing or palliating the symptoms of malignant disease in well over half of the 1.4 million diagnosed cases each year. In cooperation with a vast number of health professionals, its major focus is to promote and maintain health through treatment, research, and education.

Because this brief narrative is intended to provide an overview of the ethical and legal implications in radiation therapy, an example may prove helpful.

An insurance company was notified within 48 hours of a patient's complaint to the hospital administration that he had received less than acceptable treatment during his first week of radiation treatment for a moderately aggressive brain tumor. The radiation oncologist's prescription directed the radiation therapist to deliver a beam of external radiation to the parietal lobe of the brain from three separate angles. The radiation therapists, working in pairs to cross-check one another, were responsible for the documentation and administration of the prescribed dose of radiation therapy for Mr. Cobbs (not the patient's real name).

Mr. Cobbs became concerned after repeated small adjustments (from the perspective of the radiation therapist) were made over the first few days of treatment. He perceived these adjustments as arbitrary changes. After the third day of treatment, the daily delivery of the radiation from the anterior and left and right sides took on a more routine pattern. Only during the first few days of treatment did Mr. Cobbs suspect something was wrong. He was afraid to discuss this with the therapists because he was not sure something was actually wrong. He later shared with his wife that he could not be certain it wasn't the tumor "playing tricks on him"! The hospital's insurance company felt it was in their best interest to investigate the matter in the event a lawsuit was later filed.

The patient's specific radiation therapy records were made up of the treatment chart, including the radiation oncologist's initial consultation report; weekly treatment notes; pathology and other reports; consent forms; daily treatment records; and portal verification films (a type of x-ray examination used to check the patient's positioning, field, and block placement).

The importance of accurate record keeping is well demonstrated in this case. An independent reviewer hired by the insurance company to examine the records found them accurate and detailed. The daily treatment chart verified Mr. Cobbs's concern. During the first three days of treatment, small adjustments (less than 0.5 cm) were made in both the radiation field placement and the hand placement of shielding blocks.

Because the patient received his first treatment on the same day as the physician's consultation, hand-placed shielding blocks were used until custom-designed shielding blocks could be constructed and verified 2 days later. This perceived "change" by the patient was actually not out of the ordinary. Small adjustments and fine tuning of the treatment plan may be necessary during the initial phase of treatment, especially in a case such as Mr. Cobbs's, where treatment was initiated so soon after consultation.

Perhaps better communication among the patient, family, and therapists would have alleviated Mr. Cobbs's concerns. Good communication is essential when educating the patient. In addition to developing technical skills necessary in their practice, health care professionals must develop an understanding of informed consent, assessment, record keeping, and confidentiality.

DENNIS LEAVER, MS, RT (R) (T)
DIRECTOR, RADIATION THERAPY PROGRAM
SOUTHERN MAINE TECHNICAL COLLEGE
South Portland, Maine

CHAPTER 3

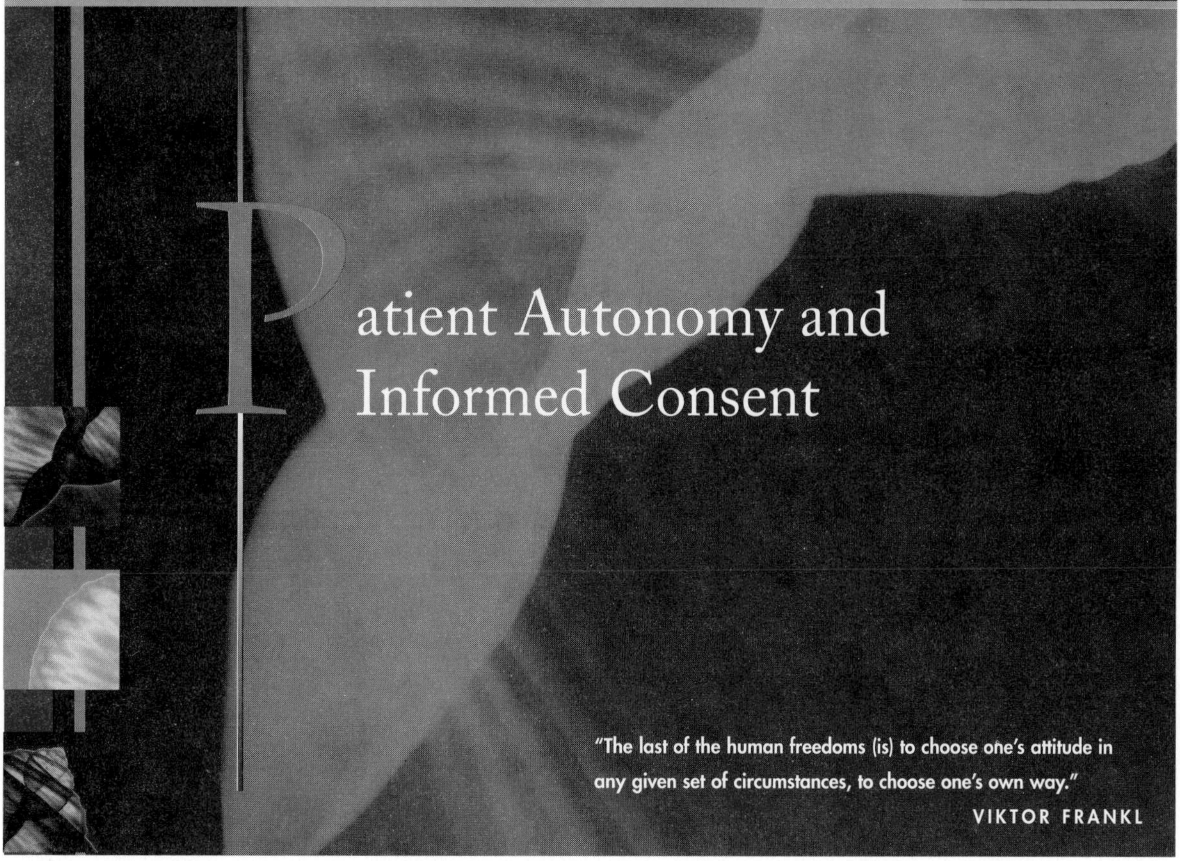

Patient Autonomy and Informed Consent

"The last of the human freedoms (is) to choose one's attitude in any given set of circumstances, to choose one's own way."

VIKTOR FRANKL

LEARNING OBJECTIVES

- Describe the relationship between autonomy and informed consent.
- Identify the stresses involved in granting informed consent and autonomy.
- Discuss methods of verifying informed consent.
- Define *surrogacy.*
- Compare and contrast competence and incompetence.
- Correlate coercion, paternalism, and therapeutic privilege.
- Explain why emergency situations and certain facilities may alter informed consent processes.
- Evaluate ethical theories that may be implemented to facilitate problem solving.
- Understand and give examples of the difference between intentional and unintentional torts and ways the perception of intent rather than the actual intent may be the basis for allegations.
- Understand and give examples of simple consent as it relates to assault, battery, and false imprisonment.
- Define informed consent, its requirements, whose duty it is, and the imaging professional's role regarding it.
- Evaluate and discuss the important but limited role of the consent form.

CHAPTER OUTLINE

ETHICAL ISSUES

Informed consent is a common concern in all the imaging modalities. Imaging professionals must be proficient in the recitation of facts and figures required to inform the patient. However, health care providers also should be able to provide patients with a process that renders them truly knowledgeable about procedures and their alternatives.

INFORMED CONSENT
Informed consent is the written assent of a patient to receive a proposed treatment; adequate information is essential for the patient to give truly informed consent.

During the early stages of development within the medical community, the patient's autonomy was not a serious consideration. Doctors were expected to be omniscient and were rarely questioned. They acted as the "fathers" of their clientele. This paternalism and the invocation of therapeutic privilege were standard professional philosophies. However, as years passed and patients became more aware of their rights and privileges, the medical community developed new methods of informing patients. The emphasis on patient autonomy and informed consent has come from many areas (Box 3-1).

AUTONOMY
Autonomy is the concept that patients are to be treated as individuals and informed about procedures to facilitate appropriate decisions.

Some physicians still find this model of patient education difficult because they believe the informational process complicates health care and brings their expertise into question. However, thankfully most physicians and institutions understand the relevance of informed consent and patients' rights.

The maintenance of patient autonomy and the obtaining of valid informed consent are vital in the vascular imaging laboratory. Imaging professionals routinely visit patients before procedures and explain the processes, contrast media involved, and physical sensations to which the patient will be subjected. They also may discuss imaging procedures with patients during transportation and preparation. These are important parts of the informational process and are vital to the maintenance of patient autonomy. Occasionally the imaging professional may be required to witness the signing of a written informed consent form. Other imaging procedures, including fluoroscopic studies and intravenous pyelograms (IVPs), often require the tech-

BOX 3-1 CRUCIAL ELEMENTS IN PATIENT AUTONOMY AND INFORMED CONSENT

- Maintenance of patients' rights
- Provision of education to facilitate consent
- Promotion of human dignity
- Determination of incompetence
- Advocacy of surrogates
- Elimination of attitudes of paternalism
- Clarification of unclear communication involving therapeutic privilege
- Strategies for dealing with emergency situations
- Use of compatible parameters for consent in specific health care facilities
- Education regarding the ethical theories involved in patient autonomy and informed consent

nologist to facilitate the informed consent process. Imaging professionals must decide whether this is appropriate using personal and professional parameters.

DEFINITION

Autonomy means "one human person, precisely as a human person, dares not have the authority and should not have power over another human person. In a medical sense, a patient will not be treated without informed consent of his or her lawful surrogates, except in narrowly defined emergencies."[1]

PATIENTS' BILL OF RIGHTS

The limits of a patient's right to information are important in considerations of autonomy. The American Hospital Association has established a Patient's Bill of Rights (See pp. 11-12).[2] The twelve points of the Bill of Rights emphasize the importance of respectful care; the right to obtain information from a physician concerning diagnosis, treatment, and prognosis in terms the patient can understand; and the right to receive information regarding risks, duration of incapacitation, alternatives, and the names of persons performing the examination before giving informed consent to any procedure. The patient also has the right to expect a hospital to respond reasonably to requests for services and continuity of service. Access to information concerning billing and costs, hospital rules and regulations, human experimentation, and relationships among the hospital and other care agencies and providers is also a patient right.[2]

The Patient's Bill of Rights outlines patient expectations and explains the way in which the process of obtaining informed consent aids the patient in obtaining these rights. The physician obtaining informed consent should describe what will happen during the procedure and any possible consequences.

INFORMATION DELIVERY

The way in which information is given depends on the criteria used to inform the patient. The following four potentially conflicting rules may guide the physician or other health care provider in explaining information to patients[1]:

1. Patient preference rule
2. Professional custom rule
3. Prudent person rule
4. Subjective substantial disclosure rule

Institutional rules also must be taken into account.

Patient Preference Rule

The patient preference rule requires health care professionals to tell patients what they want to know. For example, in the case of a patient about to undergo a procedure requiring an injection, the physician or imaging professional would say "the needle stick won't hurt."

Professional Custom Rule

The professional custom rule states that the health care professional should give the patient the information normally given to patients in similar situations. To continue the injection example, under this rule the imaging professional or physician would say "this will just be a little stick."

Prudent Person Rule

The prudent person rule, or reasonable patient standard, measures the physician's disclosure to the patient based on the patient's need for information to make decisions regarding treatment.[1] The imaging professional must consider the information the patient needs to make informed decisions concerning a procedure. In the case of the previous example, the imaging professional or physician would have to decide how much the patient needs to know about the discomfort from the needle stick before he or she can make an adequate informed consent decision.

Subjective Substantial Disclosure Rule

The subjective substantial disclosure rule encourages the physician to disseminate all information important to the individual patient. In responding to the previous example, the physician would feel obliged to explain *all* the possible ramifications of the needle stick to the patient.

The prudent person rule addresses many of the important elements of informed consent. A combination of the prudent person rule and the subjective disclosure rule, which requires the physician to communicate meaningfully with the patient, provides the information the patient needs to make an informed decision. Such a combination ensures that the physician has adequate knowledge about the patient and the patient has adequate knowledge about the procedure (Box 3-2).

Institutional Rules Regarding Informed Consent

Imaging professionals also must consider institutional rules concerning a variety of ethical issues, including informed consent. During the interview process before employment, they should investigate issues of institutional ethics and values before making choices concerning their abilities to function and provide patient care within the parameters provided by the institution.

BOX 3-2 RULES FOR EXPLAINING PROCEDURES: WHICH ONE WOULD YOU USE?

1. Patient preference rule—Provides information patients want to know
2. Professional custom rule—Provides the information normally given to patients
3. Prudent person rule—Provides the information patients need to know to consent to or refuse treatment
4. Subjective substantial disclosure rule—Provides patients with all information
5. Combination of rules—provides information without overburdening the patient

COMPLICATIONS OF AUTONOMY AND INFORMED CONSENT/RIGHT OF REFUSAL

After examining the issues included in defining patient autonomy and protecting patient rights, imaging professionals should be able to recognize the dilemmas involved in ensuring informed consent. Whether a patient may ever give truly informed consent is open to question. To be totally informed, the patient would need to be educated in many areas from anatomy to procedure. Imaging professionals may consider whether this is possible or whether informed consent is simply an idealistic (though necessary) ritual. They also must recognize their responsibility in the process of obtaining informed consent. Even if the procedure is complicated to explain, imaging professionals should make every effort to help patients become more knowledgeable. Until patients become responsible for providing and obtaining information concerning their medical procedures, a truly informed, educated consent that ensures autonomy may never be realized.

The Patient Self-Determination Act of 1991 helps ensure patient autonomy[3]:

> Heeding the principle of autonomy also means that imaging professionals should respect a patient's choice to refuse treatments. The basic human right of all patients to refuse treatment was formally legislated by the Omnibus Budget Reconciliation Act (1990). The Patient Self-Determination Act became effective December 1, 1991, and requires all health care institutions receiving Medicare or Medicaid funds to inform patients that they have the right to refuse medical and surgical care and the right to initiate a written advance directive (i.e., a written or oral statement by which a competent person makes known his or her treatment preferences and/or designates a surrogate decision maker in the event he or she should become unable to make medical decisions on his or her own behalf [Box 3-3]). Hospitals, home health care agencies, and managed care organizations are required to make this information available, in writing, at the time the patient comes under an agency's care.

BOX 3-3 REQUIREMENTS OF THE PATIENT SELF-DETERMINATION ACT

- Provision of written information to adult patients about their rights to make medical decisions, including the right to accept or refuse treatment and the right to formulate advance directives
- Documentation in each patient's record regarding whether the patient has executed an advance directive
- Implementation of written policies regarding the various types of advance directives
- Ensuring of compliance with state laws regarding medical treatment decisions and advance directives
- Elimination of discrimination against individuals regarding their treatment decisions made through an advance directive
- Provision of education for staff members and the community on ethical and legal issues concerning advance directives

From the Omnibus Budget Reconciliation Act of 1990, Sections 4206 and 4751, Public Law 101-508, November 5, 1990.

VERIFICATION OF INFORMED CONSENT

One ethical challenge inherent in many imaging procedures is the appropriateness of the verification of informed consent. Imaging professionals should always be available to answer questions that patients may have concerning their procedures. However, questions concerning specifics of informed consent such as alternative therapies, contrast reactions, failure rate, risks, or other subjects should always be directed to the patient's physician.

The physician has a crucial role in the process of obtaining informed consent. Because of their knowledge and expertise, physicians bear the responsibility for informing patients concerning procedures. The imaging professional should refer the patient to the physician concerning questions about the procedure to facilitate the informed consent process.

Another important ethical consideration is whether imaging professionals should allow themselves to be placed in the position of witnessing the patient's signature on the informed consent form. Imaging professionals commonly are given the responsibility for getting the patient to sign the imaging procedure consent form. If they are not present when the patient's physician presumably gives the necessary instructions and explanations to the patient, they are only qualified to witness the fact that the patient has signed the form. If litigation were to occur, the imaging professional could not attest to the fact that the patient gave informed consent, only that the patient signed the form.

Many imaging professionals involved in carrying out informed consent procedures find themselves in the difficult situation of determining how much of the responsibility for informed consent is theirs. Nevertheless, few have probably even questioned this process. Many student imaging professionals are required to explain the injection of contrast media and possible reactions to patients as part of their clinical objectives. Although these students must learn this skill, imaging professionals may need to consider whether this important educational duty should be left to students and whether this is conducive to the patient's truly informed consent and the imaging professional's protection from liability.

An example of the difficulties inherent in ensuring patient autonomy and eliciting truly informed consent may be observed in a fluoroscopic imaging suite in which gastrointestinal procedures are performed. The patient may have been informed, but can anyone ever be ready for an air contrast colon examination? Patients subjected to this procedure are already afraid, sick, and in pain and may feel as though they have no control over their care. Imaging professionals need to consider ways of facing this challenge and informing patients as fully as possible about an often dehumanizing procedure without completely discouraging them from an examination that may have enormous diagnostic benefits. Throughout all of this, the dignity and autonomy of the patient must be preserved.

An imaging professional may overhear a co-worker speaking disrespectfully about a patient who is unconscious or deaf. Because respect for freedom and privacy is ultimately rooted in the dignity of each person, the maintenance of autonomy requires health care providers to respect all individuals, even those who are not currently capable of free choice.[1] In short, people do not lose their dignity because they are unconscious, in a coma, or out of contact with reality. Such patients present special difficulties, but they must nevertheless be respected. Dignity and autonomy do not stem from a person's ability to function in an imaging suite; instead, the clinical area should accommodate itself to the individual's limitations.

COMPETENCE AND INCOMPETENCE SURROGACY

COMPETENCE
Competence is the ability to make choices.

Competence is a necessary element in informed consent. In the medical setting, competence entails the ability to make appropriate choices and consider their consequences. A patient's competence may be temporarily compromised by prescription or over-the-counter drugs. In this condition of short-term incompetence, the patient may require a surrogate or the procedure may need to be postponed until the patient is competent. Proving incompetence is difficult. An evaluation of the patient's ability to make decisions is an important component in determining competence.

Imaging professionals need to consider the ways in which they deal with patients who are temporarily incompetent or rendered permanently incompetent by brain damage, developmental disabilities, dementia, or Alzheimer's disease. Such patients do not have less dignity or less of a right to be informed. Even the most incompetent person has basic human dignity, and imaging professionals must keep this in mind.

Questions regarding methods for determining competence and adequately informing patients who are incompetent often lead to a consideration of surrogacy, or the appointment of a person or persons to make decisions regarding care in the name of the patient. A surrogate may be a parent, an individual named by the patient while competent, or a person or persons appointed by the courts. Surrogates may be involved in the determination of competence and in the informed consent process. As such, they may pose an obstacle to autonomy, especially if the patient gave no advance directives regarding personal wishes. No person can ever truly know the wishes of another; nevertheless, surrogates must do their best to surmise the patient's wishes.

OBSTACLES TO AUTONOMY AND INFORMED CONSENT

Other hindrances to autonomy include undue influences that may restrict the patient's choices. Ill patients may feel pressured into decisions as a result of concern for their health, future, and family members. Imaging professionals must be careful not to add any other influences that may render patients, who have already experienced a loss of personal freedom, unable to make decisions concerning their care. The imaging suite environment itself may negatively influence the patient; its intimidating atmosphere may frighten the patient past the point of sound decision making. Imaging professionals must therefore make every effort to calm and reassure the patient. At the same time, they should recognize that no person is ever completely free from outside influences and as such truly informed, educated consent and autonomy may be impossible.

The patient's family members or physician may pressure the patient because of personal or professional feelings concerning the patient's welfare. Lack of communication on the part of the patient or professional also may interfere with the informed consent process. In this situation the professional should receive feedback from the patient to verify that the information was understood.

Serious obstacles to autonomy and informed consent may spring from health care providers, including physicians, nurses, and allied health professionals. Because of their education and experience, they often believe they know what is best for patients. They are then confused and sometimes angry when patients refuse treatment or question their explanations. This attitude of paternalism is unhealthy for autonomy. Patients may perceive these attitudes on the part of the provider, which may reinforce any distrust they may already have had. An irritated, know-it-all imaging professional may frighten or annoy a patient out of the examination room and past the point of diagnosis. Clear communication between the provider and patient is crucial, and the imaging professional has an obligation to communicate properly and not merely spout facts. If the patient does not understand, informed consent is not possible. Imaging professionals should remember to talk *to* patients, not *at* them.

Imaging professionals may become so accustomed to the repetition of information that they do not truly listen to patients. Students especially may be so involved in covering all the information that they sound like waiters explaining the catch of the day, not professionals describing the possible complications of a medical procedure. Patients are usually frightened, and when asked if they understand, may nod "yes" with heads empty of understanding.

THERAPEUTIC PRIVILEGE

Physicians and imaging professionals must decide what the patient needs to know; these difficult decisions usually raise the issue of therapeutic privilege, a prerogative invoked when health care providers withhold information from patients because they believe the information would have adverse effects on the patients' conditions or health. Physicians and other health care providers may believe they are knowledgeable about what the patient can tolerate. They may use this belief as a reason to omit information if they believe it may have adverse effects on patients. Imaging professionals who believe they know the way patients feel better than they do should reevaluate their omission of information. Therapeutic privilege is used less often by caregivers who realize that patients are becoming much more aware of their rights. When their autonomy is denied, their ability to give informed consent is impaired. Most patients want to be told the truth about their conditions. When imaging professionals omit necessary information, the result may be deceit, mistrust, and very possibly harm to the patient.

EMERGENCY SITUATIONS

Certain facilities and situations may pose serious threats to autonomy and informed consent. Mental health facilities and nursing homes may compromise the autonomy processes. Many patients in these institutions are considered incompetent as a result of mental illness or age, although neither of these factors necessarily renders

ADVANCE DIRECTIVE
An advance directive is a predetermined (usually written) choice made to inform others of the ways in which the patient wishes to be treated while incompetent.

the patient incompetent. Many mental health and nursing facilities are now asking competent patients to give written advance directives or assign a surrogate to provide protection for the patient and provider if the patient becomes incompetent at a later date.

In emergency situations the informed consent process may need to be abandoned to save the patient's life. Imaging professionals may find themselves in such situations in the emergency department. According to the laws of many states, three conditions must be present for the omission of informed consent to be justified:

1. The patient must be incapable of giving consent and no lawful surrogate is available.
2. Danger to life or risk of a serious impairment to health is apparent.
3. Immediate treatment is necessary to avert these dangers.

Providing treatment without the patient's consent may be considered a denial of autonomy; however, autonomy is not relevant if the patient dies. In this case, autonomy becomes a consideration of the patient's family or surrogate. If the family feels the patient's rights have been denied, they may take legal action. Many emergency room physicians are faced with this difficult situation and the quick but vital decisions it requires. Informed consent and autonomy are not always possible in emergency situations. In life-and-death situations, if the patient is unable to comprehend or communicate and a surrogate is unavailable, emergency treatment is always appropriate.

APPLICATION OF ETHICAL THEORIES TO AUTONOMY

The imaging professional may experience further difficulty in choosing a theory of ethics to apply when considering patient autonomy. The theory of consequentialism (utilitarianism) requires the greatest good to be done for the greatest number. Deontology holds that the motives for an action are the most important considerations. Virtue ethics invokes practical wisdom and right reason. (See Chapter 1 for a more detailed review of ethical theories.)

Utilitarianism is not very relevant in considerations of autonomy and consent because it generally is applied to large numbers of persons. Although the informed consent process may affect other persons, the patient has a more immediate interest in understanding the process. The deontologic viewpoint, with its emphasis on motives instead of consequences, is difficult to apply in considerations of the maintenance of a patient's autonomy because in this situation, the consequences are crucial. Both utilitarianism and deontology assume that people use ethical constructs to address the difficulties involved in encouraging the individual's autonomy while obtaining genuinely informed consent. However, because moral significance and other factors vary with each individual, even those using similar constructs may come to differing conclusions.

Virtue ethics relies on virtues, practical wisdom, and an appreciation of the consequences of actions. This theory is the most adaptable for dealing with the difficulties of patient autonomy because it promotes the dignity of patients and their freedom of choice.

IMAGING SCENARIO

A 90-year-old patient with terminal cancer who is mentally limited, hard of hearing, and visually impaired is scheduled for an enteroclysis. Even a healthy 20-year-old patient may have difficulty with this procedure, which is embarrassing and often painful. The imaging professional wonders why this terminally ill, feeble, geriatric patient should be forced to endure this procedure. Does the patient truly understand what it entails? The patient may have been influenced by a physician concerned with doing everything possible to avoid legal repercussions, and informed consent may have been given by a family member who wants to hang on to Granddad no matter what. If the patient had made himself clearer concerning his wishes before the illness became invasive, all the involved parties would not be struggling with the implications and consequences of the procedure. In what way do the three ethical theories address the difficult decisions involved in this scenario?

LEGAL ISSUES

Patient autonomy is crucial to many legal theories applicable to imaging professionals. Consent and informed consent are the two legal issues in which patient autonomy is most obvious and necessary. Failure to obtain consent may result in allegations of torts such as assault, battery, false imprisonment, and negligence with regard to lack of informed consent.

These torts are discussed in this chapter. Legal issues regarding consent, informed consent, and the imaging professional's role in both are discussed at length in this chapter.

TORT LAW

A tort is a civil wrong for which the law provides a remedy.[4] A tort action is filed to recover damages for personal injury or property damage occurring from negligent conduct or intentional misconduct. Tort law may be divided into two categories—intentional torts and unintentional torts. Intentional torts result when an act is done with the intention of causing harm to another.[4] The intentional torts that are most likely to have an impact on the provision of medical imaging services are assault, battery, false imprisonment, and defamation. Assault, battery, and false imprisonment are discussed in this chapter. Defamation is discussed in Chapter 4, which covers truthfulness and confidentiality.

Simple Consent

Justice Cordoza stated in the 1914 *Scloendoff* case[5] that "every human being of adult years and sound mind has a right to determine what shall be done with his own body; and a surgeon who performs an operation without his consent commits an assault for which he is liable in damages." This court decision provided the basis for the concept of consent and established that violation of consent constitutes assault and battery.

SIMPLE CONSENT
Simple consent is the assent required of a patient for any procedure.

A patient must consent to any procedure. This simple consent does not require knowledge of the procedure. It simply means that a patient's permission must be obtained before the procedure can be performed. Consent may be given simply by the patient getting on the table or stepping up to the chest board. If a patient is in an emergency situation, consent need not be asked for or given. Instead, the situation is evaluated legally by assessing what a reasonable person would do in a similar situation. Again, the applicable standard of care prevails.

Most problems with simple consent arise when consent is withdrawn by a patient or if the boundaries of what that patient has consented to are exceeded. This may be a difficult situation to address, because although an imaging professional cannot continue a procedure without the patient's consent, the patient often may be reassured by a more thorough explanation of the procedure, and consent can again be obtained.

Intentional Torts

Although the concept of a provider of medical imaging services intending to harm a patient is bizarre, if the patient feels the tort was intended, the determination of intent may well be left to a jury. Communication with patients to ensure patient understanding is the best tool to lessen or decrease the risk of allegations of intentional torts.

INTENTIONAL TORTS
Intentional torts are wrongs resulting from acts done with the intention of causing harm to another.

ASSAULT
Assault is a deliberate act wherein one person threatens to harm another without consent and the victim feels the attacker has the ability to carry out the threat.

BATTERY
Battery is touching to which the victim has not consented.

Assault and Battery

An assault is a deliberate act wherein one person threatens to harm another person without consent and the victim perceives that the other has the ability to carry out the threat.[6] Battery is touching to which the victim has not consented, even if the touching may benefit the patient.[6] For example, assault may be alleged if an imaging professional threatens to perform a portable chest x-ray examination on a competent person against his or her will. Battery occurs if the x-ray examination is actually performed on the competent, unwilling patient.

In situations involving patients who are incompetent or those requiring restraint, the law allows providers to touch patients without consent. In these situations, consideration must be given to four important conditions (Box 3-4).

Although restraints are commonly used in the medical imaging department, imaging professionals must keep in mind that they should be able to justify use of restraints

BOX 3-4 LEGAL CRITERIA FOR THE USE OF RESTRAINT

1. Touching or restraint to which the patient has not consented is needed to protect the patient, health care team members, or the property of others.
2. The restraint used is the least intrusive method possible.
3. Regular reassessment of the need to restrain occurs.
4. The restraint is discontinued as soon as practicable.

Modified from Harper F, James F, Gray O: *The law of torts,* ed 3, Boston, 1996, Little, Brown & Company.

according to the four criteria listed in Box 3-4. When dealing with children, imaging technologists must communicate clearly with parents. This communication not only increases parental confidence in the imaging professionals but also minimizes the risk of litigation. Adequate communication should include an explanation of the necessity for restraint to decrease radiation exposure and obtain optimal studies, reassurance that the restraint equipment used is the least intrusive, and a guarantee it will be used only when necessary and discontinued as soon as possible.

False Imprisonment

Although false imprisonment seems to be a ridiculous allegation to make against an imaging professional, certain circumstances in the medical imaging setting may give rise to such allegations. False imprisonment occurs when a person is unlawfully confined within a fixed area.[6] The confined person must be aware of the confinement or must be harmed by the confinement. Additionally, even if the person is not actually confined, if the perception is one of confinement (e.g., the patient thinks he is in a locked imaging room, even though the door is not locked), the possibility of this allegation exists.[6]

FALSE IMPRISONMENT
False imprisonment is the unlawful confinement of a person within a fixed area.

For false imprisonment to be found, plaintiffs must prove they were restrained either physically or by threat or intimidation and that they did not consent to the restraint.[6] Because restraints are often important and necessary tools in obtaining successful medical images or therapeutic treatment, a successful false imprisonment suit requires the jury to find that an imaging professional acted in an unreasonable, unjustified, and unprivileged manner.[6] Again, the applicable standard of care is used.

Damages recoverable for false imprisonment include compensation for bodily injury, physical discomfort, inconvenience, loss of time and wages, emotional distress, harm to reputation, and the loss of company of one's family.[6] If the imprisonment is extremely outrageous, punitive damages also may be awarded.[7]

Unintentional Torts

Unintentional torts result from actions that were not intended to cause harm. The unintentional tort most commonly encountered in medical imaging is medical malpractice, a broad term that in most jurisdictions encompasses negligence, failure to obtain informed consent, and breach of patient confidentiality. All these causes of action are alleged based on the fact that a duty is owed, the duty is breached, and harm results from the breach.

UNINTENTIONAL TORTS
Unintentional torts are wrongs resulting from actions that were not intended to do harm.

In the health care setting, duties are owed to patients by physicians, hospitals or other health care facilities, and all health care providers, including imaging professionals. If a duty is not performed adequately, in violation of a statute or as judged by the appropriate standard of care, and harm results from the failure to perform the duty adequately, liability may be found.

Medical negligence was discussed in Chapter 2, and breach of confidentiality is discussed in Chapter 4. Medical malpractice cases alleging failure to obtain informed consent are discussed here because patient autonomy is the ethical principle underpinning informed consent.

Informed Consent

Case law concerning informed consent was established in the 1957 case of *Salgo v Leland and the Stanford University Board of Trustees*[8] and the 1972 case of *Canterbury v Spence.*[9] These cases established that the physician has a legal duty to obtain consent. They further required physicians to give patients enough information regarding risks, benefits, alternative treatment options, and expected outcomes if they chose not to undergo the proposed diagnostic testing or treatment to enable them to make informed decisions.

According to the *Canterbury* case, informed consent is necessary to allow the patient to determine the direction of treatment.[9] The amount of information needed for this determination varies depending on the patient and the procedure. Physicians must use their medical knowledge and experience to determine the information a reasonable person needs to make an informed and intelligent decision.[9] Generally, the physician is required to describe the benefits of the procedure and the accompanying risks, including the risk of death or paralysis.[10]

Two basic exceptions exist in which informed consent need not be obtained—emergency situations and cases in which therapeutic privilege is invoked. The emergency exception occurs only if the patient is unconscious or otherwise unable to give consent, and harm from failure to treat is imminent and outweighs any harm inherent in the proposed treatment. Therapeutic privilege applies only if risk disclosure poses such a threat to the patient that it will lead to further harm. The physician must have reason to believe that the patient would become unusually emotionally distraught if the information were disclosed.[9]

To prove lack of informed consent, a plaintiff must prove a material risk existed that was unknown to the patient, the risk was not disclosed, disclosure of the risk would have led a reasonable patient to reject the medical procedure or choose a different course of treatment, and the patient was injured as a result of the lack of disclosure.[11]

Case law regarding informed consent has been discussed. Statutes can also regulate informed consent procedures, and in many states, statutes have established panels that determine which procedures require written informed consent and define exactly what must be disclosed, including the wording to be used. Additionally, facilities and physicians are free to establish more stringent requirements of disclosure for patients.

Liability is often not found because the jury cannot determine that a reasonable patient who had been informed would have rejected the procedure. Whether or not liability is imposed on this basis, a great deal of time (on the part of lawyers, employees, and physicians), money, and emotional distress is expended in litigation. Therefore, consistently obtaining informed consent is a valuable risk management tool.

Case Studies

The following cases demonstrate the legal issues inherent in informed consent. The 1987 Iowa Supreme Court decision in *Pauscher v Iowa Methodist Medical Center* clarified the elements necessary to prove lack of informed consent.

Becky Pauscher was scheduled for an IVP 6 days after delivering her first child because of fever, pain in her right side, and blood in her urine. No physician told Mrs. Pauscher that severe reactions to the procedure included the possibility of death, nor did anyone ask if Mrs. Pauscher consented to the procedure. The requisition could not be found after the procedure, but the technologist stated that Mrs. Pauscher had denied allergies. Her chart, however, noted an allergy to bee stings and a history of asthma as a child.

After the injection of some of the contrast medium, Mrs. Pauscher began to scratch her face. The technologist stopped the injection, but continued after seeing no further distress signs. When Mrs. Pauscher complained of chest pain, the technologist again stopped the injection and called the radiologist. Mrs. Pauscher died of anaphylactic shock despite resuscitation attempts.

Mrs. Pauscher's husband sued the urologist and radiologist for failing to disclose the risk of death, stating his wife could not make an informed choice without that knowledge. He charged the hospital with failing to have an established policy for informed consent.

The Iowa Supreme Court found that the physicians were responsible for informing the patient of the risks, but determined Mrs. Pauscher would not have refused the test based on the "extremely remote" risk of death.

The Pauscher case did not find the hospital to have a duty to inform the patient of risks nor obtain informed consent. This is generally the state of the law regarding informed consent. However, such a duty has been recognized in at least one jurisdiction.

The 1992 Kentucky Supreme Court case of *Keel v St. Elizabeth Medical Center* found the hospital liable for failure to obtain informed consent.[12] In this case, Leslie Keel came to the St. Elizabeth Medical Center for a computed tomography (CT) scan with contrast injection. Before the test, Mr. Keel was given no information concerning risks. Whether Mr. Keel responded to questions regarding allergies and previous history of reactions to contrast injections is uncertain. Mr. Keel later developed a thrombophlebitis at the injection site.

This court separated the issue of informed consent from the issue of negligence. Although the issue of whether the injection was negligently performed was not explored, the court found the hospital had a statutory duty to disclose the risks of the procedure and failed to perform that duty.

Case law in other jurisdictions indicates a refusal to impose a duty on hospitals to inform patients of the material risks of a procedure prescribed by the patient's physician and to obtain informed consent. Some of these courts refused to find such a duty for a hospital based on statutes that impose this duty only on the physician.[15] Other courts followed previous authority in refusing to find such a duty for hospitals.[16] *Goss v Oklahoma Blood Institute* cited authority from Washington, Iowa, Florida, Texas, North Carolina, New Mexico, North Dakota, Colorado, Michigan, West Virginia, and Illinois for support in its refusal to recognize a duty for the hospital to disclose risks and obtain informed consent.[17]

Generally, the duty to obtain informed consent is the physician's. However, because the law varies by jurisdiction, imaging professionals should be aware of the law in their particular jurisdictions.

BOX 3-5 ELEMENTS IN INFORMED CONSENT

- The consent must be given voluntarily by a mentally competent adult. The patient should not be coerced into giving consent.
- Patients must understand exactly to what they are consenting. If a patient speaks a foreign language or is deaf, an interpreter must explain the procedure requiring consent.
- The request for consent should include a description of the risks and benefits of the procedure, alternative treatment options, and expected outcomes if treatment is not commenced.
- The consent should be written, signed by the patient or representative, witnessed, and dated.
- Consent to treat a minor patient usually is given by a parent or guardian, but if the minor patient is at least 7 years old, he or she should be included in the decision-making process.

Modified from Deloughery GL: Key elements for informed consent. In Deloughery GL, editor: *Issues and trends in nursing,* St Louis, 1995, Mosby.

Obtaining Valid Informed Consent

The patient's capacity to consent to or refuse the procedure must be evaluated. The primary issue to be considered is whether the patient is capable of understanding the medical condition and the risks, benefits, alternative treatment options, and expected outcomes if treatment is not commenced (Box 3-5).

Although the physician bears the ultimate responsibility for obtaining valid informed consent, imaging professionals often must make subjective judgments of patients' capacities to make decisions. This is particularly true if the patient is in severe pain.

If imaging professionals, after consulting with radiologists, do not feel that patients have the capacity to give valid informed consent, they should seek surrogate consent. If such consent is impossible to obtain, the involved parties should consider invoking the emergency exception to the informed consent doctrine. If that exception does not apply, the procedure should not be performed.

Patients who are minors are another problematic population for informed consent. Historically, consent was obtained on behalf of a minor by a parent or guardian (most states define *minor* as a person less than 18 years of age). However, with the advent of cases such as the 1992 case of Gregory K., in which a minor sued his mother for divorce, courts are allowing minors more rights in the decision-making process.[16]

Inclusion of the minor patient in the decision-making process is advisable because it allows the minor to indicate a difference of opinion from the parents. If a conflict develops between the wishes of the two parties, the imaging professional should seek help from the hospital's legal counsel to determine the law in that jurisdiction.

Role of Imaging Professionals in Informed Consent

As has been discussed, informed consent is absolutely necessary. Although legal responsibility for obtaining consent lies with the physician, most facilities have adopted policies and procedures also requiring imaging professionals to ensure that informed consent is obtained. Imaging professionals should recognize this responsibility as part of any procedure requiring written consent they perform. Because imaging professionals are the people performing the study, they have a duty to ensure that procedures are explained and consent obtained before beginning the procedure.

Imaging professionals have excellent opportunities to explain procedures to patients. They spend much more time with patients than do physicians, and their communication with patients helps build a good imaging professional/patient relationship that not only makes the patient more comfortable about asking questions concerning the procedure but also is more likely to result in a better outcome.

Consent Forms

Forms are useful tools to help inform patients about procedures and document consent. A single form adapted to include specifics of the particular procedure requiring consent or multiple forms specifically designed for each procedure may be used. Because each state and facility has different legal requirements, these forms should be carefully written with input from physicians, the technologists performing the studies, risk management, and legal counsel.[17]

The forms should be written clearly in terms understandable by laypersons and must be used in conjunction with a thorough explanation to the patient that includes a discussion of risks, benefits, alternative diagnostic or treatment plans, and expected outcomes if the patient decides not to undergo the procedure. A consent form must never be used in place of an oral explanation.

CONSENT FORMS
Consent forms are useful tools to help inform patients about procedures and document consent.

Generally, a consent form includes the name of the procedure; a brief explanation of the procedure, including benefits and risks; spaces for the patient's name and the name of the person performing the procedure; and signature lines for the

IMAGING SCENARIO

The imaging department is swamped and you find yourself relieving an imaging professional in the IVP room. He tells you everything is ready for you to inject the patient. You speak to the radiologist between other procedures and she hurriedly comes in and injects the contrast without inquiring about informed consent or looking at the form. Just as you finish the IVP films, the patient starts to exhibit signs of anaphylactic shock. The appropriate emergency care is administered, but the patient ends up in intensive care and eventually dies, leaving behind a husband and a 3-month-old child. As the activity in the IVP room dies down, you notice that the informed consent form is neither filled out nor signed.

Discussion questions

- Have you created liability for yourself?
- Have you created liability for the hospital?
- Have you created liability for the radiologist?
- What must the family prove to be successful in a lawsuit?

patient or surrogate, the person explaining the procedure and obtaining consent, and at least one witness.[14] The form also must be dated with the time recorded. Laws and facility regulations vary, but in general consent should be obtained within 24 hours before the procedure.

Policies and procedures should be developed regarding when written consent must be obtained. They should ensure that consent is obtained in writing whenever an invasive procedure is performed or when a procedure has associated risks and disclosure of these risks may be helpful to a patient in deciding whether to undergo the procedure. If informed consent forms are computerized, these forms and their accompanying patient signatures should become part of the permanent patient record.

SUMMARY

The informed consent process seeks to provide the patient with enough information to facilitate the making of informed decisions concerning whether to undergo certain medical procedures. This consent process enables the patient to maintain dignity, independence, and autonomy. Physicians and other professionals attempting to obtain informed consent should provide patients with information concerning diagnosis, treatment, prognosis, risks, duration of incapacitation, alternatives, billing costs, hospital rules, and the names of persons performing the procedure.

Four rules that provide the patient with information to make an informed decision are the patient preference rule, prudent person rule, subjective substantial disclosure rule, and the professional custom rule. The prudent person rule, which discloses information the patient needs to know to decide or refuse treatment, and the subjective substantial disclosure rule, which dictates all information concerning the examination be given, are a good combination to use in the informed consent process.

Competence is necessary and a key concept in giving informed consent. If the patient is incompetent, an advance directive or surrogate may aid the process.

Obstacles to autonomy and informed consent include undue influence on patients, paternalism, therapeutic privilege, and inept communication.

Emergency situations may necessitate dispensing with informed consent processes in order to save the patient's life. Informed consent also may be superseded by therapeutic privilege if the physician feels the disclosure would cause the patient to become unusually emotionally distraught. However, this privilege should only be invoked in rare circumstances.

The theories of consequentialism, deontology, or virtue ethics may be employed to give informed consent and ensure autonomy. Virtue ethics, involving practical wisdom and reason, may be effective when dealing with issues of competence, surrogacy, obstacles to autonomy, and emergency situations.

In the future, patient autonomy will become a more expected application of medical ethics because of the changing roles and attitudes of patients and care givers; however, the achievement of absolute patient autonomy and informed consent may be impossible. As society becomes more involved in the education processes of health care and individuals become more involved in all aspects of their health care, the maintenance of patient autonomy may become a more readily achievable goal.

Patient autonomy is the ethical theory behind issues of consent and informed consent. Failure to obtain consent can result in allegations of assault, battery, or false imprisonment. Assault, battery, and false imprisonment are intentional torts, meaning the acts are done with the intent of harming another. This intent can be considered by a jury if a patient alleges that he or she perceived the act to be intentional.

Assault is a deliberate act wherein one person threatens to harm another without his or her consent and it appears that he or she has the ability to carry out the act. A battery occurs when a person is touched without giving consent. Patient consent is critical in minimizing the risks of these torts. False imprisonment is another intentional tort that occurs when a person is restrained unlawfully without giving consent. If the patient perceives that he or she is confined, even if this is not true, these allegations may be made.

Issues of restraint in the role of imaging professionals come to mind in consideration of these torts. When restraints are necessary, the imaging professional must be able to justify that restraint using the following criteria:

- Is the restraint necessary to protect the patient, health care team members, or the property of others?
- Is the restraint used the least intrusive method possible?
- Is there regular reassessment of the need to restrain?
- Is the restraint discontinued as soon as practicable?

Communication is the best tool imaging professionals have to prevent allegations of these torts. Obtaining consent and explaining necessary restraints to patients and parents limits the risk of these allegations.

Unintentional torts, which result from acts not intended to cause harm, include negligence, lack of informed consent, and breach of patient confidentiality. (Negligence is discussed in Chapter 2 and breach of confidentiality is discussed in Chapter 4.) Informed consent is required for invasive procedures and those for which disclosure of associated risks is beneficial to the patient in determining whether to proceed with the procedure or treatment.

The physician has the legal duty to obtain informed consent. However, many facilities require the imaging professional to ensure that informed consent is obtained and the proper documentation is made on the patient's chart. During preparation for the procedure, imaging professionals can talk with patients to encourage communication and gauge understanding.

Consent forms are helpful to inform patients about procedures and document consent. These forms, however, cannot substitute for the required explanation of the procedure and disclosure of associated risks. Case law has established that full disclosure requires the physician to give the patient enough information, including a discussion of the risks, benefits, alternative treatment options, and expected outcomes if the patient does not undergo the proposed treatment, to enable an informed decision about the proposed treatment.

The goal of informed consent is to allow patients to make determinations regarding the direction of their treatment. Physicians must use their medical knowledge and experience to determine how much information a reasonable patient needs to make this determination.

Policies and procedures should be in place defining when written informed consent is needed. The imaging professional's role is to be aware of procedures requiring informed consent and consistently monitor whether informed consent is obtained and documented in the patient's chart.

ENDNOTES

1. Garrett TM, Baillie HW, Garrett RM: *Healthcare ethics, principles and problems,* ed 2, Englewood Cliffs, NJ, 1993, Prentice Hall.
2. American Hospital Association: *A patient's bill of rights,* Chicago, 1992, Author.
3. Mezey M et al: The patient self-determination act: sources of concern for nurses, *Nurs Outlook* 42(1):30, 1994.
4. Prosser W, Wade J, Schwartz V: *Cases and materials on torts,* ed 8, Westbury, NY, 1988, Foundation Press.
5. *Scloendoff v Society of NY Hospitals,* 105 N.E.92 (NY 1914).
6. Harper F, James F, Gray O: *The law of torts,* ed 3, Boston, 1996, Little, Brown & Company.
7. *Dick v Watonwan County,* 562 F. Supp.1083 (D. Minn. 1983); rev'd other grounds, 738 F.2d 939 (8th Cir. 1989).
8. *Salgo v Leland and the Stanford University Board of Trustees* (Cal. 1957).
9. *Canterbury v Spence,* 464 F.2d 772 (1972).
10. *Truman v Thomas,* 611 P.2d 902 (Cal. 1980).
11. *Pauscher v Iowa Methodist Medical Center, Watter, and Bardole,* 408N.W.2d 355 (Iowa, 1987).
12. *Keel v St. Elizabeth Medical Center,* 842 S.W.2d 860 (Ky. 1992).
13. Wingert P, Salholz E: Irreconcilable differences, *Newsweek,* Sept 21, 1992.
14. Obergfell A: *Law & ethics in diagnostic imaging and therapeutic radiology,* Philadelphia, 1995, Saunders.
15. *Boney v Mother Frances Hospital,* 880 S.W.2d 140 (Tex. App.—Tyler 1994); *Kelley v Kitahama,* 675 So.2d 1181 (La. App. 5 Cir. 1996).
16. *Jones v Philadelphia College of Osteopathic Medicine,* 813 F. Supp. 1125 (E.D.Pa. 1993); *Goss v Oklahoma Blood Institute,* 856 P.2d 998 (Okl. App. 1990); *Johnson v Sears, Roebuck, & Company,* 832 P.2d 797 (N.M. App. 1992); *Winters v Podzamsky,* 621 N.E.2d 72 (Ill. App. 3 Dist. 1993).
17. *Goss v Oklahoma Blood Institute,* 856 P.2d 998 (Okl. App. 1990).

REVIEW QUESTIONS

1 Autonomy involves which of the following?
   a. Informed consent
   b. The self
   c. Patient rights
   d. All the above

2 Informed consent should include the following:
   a. ______________
   b. ______________
   c. ______________
   d. ______________

3 Why is two-way communication between patients and imaging professionals important in imaging services?

4 Should the imaging professional be responsible for the informed consent process? Explain.

5 Define the following terms:
   Competence
   Surrogacy

6 *Paternalism* is defined as which of the following?
   a. Motherlike care taking
   b. Fatherlike (Godlike) care taking
   c. Necessary
   d. None of the above

7 Define *therapeutic privilege.*

8 Describe three conditions in which emergency situations may alter the informed consent process:
   a. ______________
   b. ______________
   c. ______________

9 **True or False** Combining the prudent person rule and the subjective substantial disclosure rule in most cases provides the information the patient needs to make informed decisions.

10 **True or False** Truly informed consent may not be possible.

11 **True or False** Intentional torts can occur only if the perpetrator of the tort intends to do harm.

12 **True or False** Assault occurs when the victim is touched without giving consent.

13 **True or False** Battery cannot be found if the touching to which the patient has not consented is for the good of the patient.

14 **True or False** Restraint of patients by imaging professionals is always an exception to the torts of assault and battery.

15 **True or False** Communication is the imaging professional's best tool to decrease risk of litigation for assault, battery, and false imprisonment.

16 **True or False** The legal duty to obtain informed consent lies with the imaging professional.
17 **True or False** Informed consent need not be given if an imaging professional does not feel the patient wants to know about the procedure.
18 **True or False** The duty of informed consent lies with physicians, so imaging professionals do not need to concern themselves.
19 **True or False** Consent forms may be used to obtain consent instead of an explanation of the procedure and its risks.

CRITICAL THINKING QUESTIONS & ACTIVITIES

1 Is everyone in every situation entitled to autonomy in an imaging procedure? Why or why not?
2 What would you do in a critical situation if the patient were unresponsive and a surrogate was not available?
3 What would you do if you made the best decision you could in question 2 and were still involved in a lawsuit?
4 In what ways can imaging professionals promote the autonomy of patients in the imaging department?
5 Does the imaging professional's autonomy enhance or interfere with patient autonomy? In what way does this occur?
6 A 79-year-old female patient arrives with severe chest pain and breathlessness. She has been treated previously for a minor stroke and had a breast removed 4 years ago. She is a nervous individual and does not want to deal with decision making; she would much rather have the physician make the decision concerning a cardiac catheterization. Her family wants her to proceed with the catheterization and consider surgery. She continues to fear the process and refuses to make a decision.

Role play the various processes that may occur in this particular informed consent process and indicate ways of encouraging autonomy for the fearful patient (by one or more groups of players). As the situation is played, the observers should record the appropriate and inappropriate methods employed. These could include any of the following:

1. Positive and negative methods for obtaining informed consent and delivering information
2. Attempts to ensure autonomy
3. Paternalism
4. Invocation of therapeutic privilege
5. Surrogacy
6. Responses to emergency situations

Include these elements in your evaluation.

CRITICAL THINKING QUESTIONS & ACTIVITIES—cont'd

7 Discuss whether a person who commits an intentional tort must have the intent to cause harm to be liable.

8 Discuss situations that may result in allegations of assault or battery.

9 Discuss whether a patient can feel imprisoned without consent in the imaging department.

10 Discuss the ways in which restraints may be used and justified by the criteria presented in this chapter.

11 Discuss situations in which the imaging professional is in a difficult situation because the radiologist or interpreting physician does not want to take the time to inform the patient adequately about risks, alternative procedures, and expected outcomes if the procedure is not performed.

PROFESSIONAL PROFILE

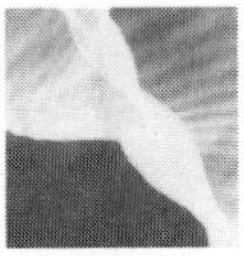

A SONOGRAPHER in a busy hospital radiology department performed survey obstetric sonograms before the performance of amniocentesis procedures. She localized a preliminary site and requested that the radiologist come in and verify the amniocentesis site. The sonographer read several of the reports regarding the amniocentesis localization procedures and noticed that the radiologist dictated that the site was selected by the sonographer and included her name in the report.

During the amniocentesis procedure, the radiologist came into the room, but would offer no advice to the obstetrician regarding the accuracy of the selected site. The rate of multiple sticks during amniocentesis procedures as well as the morbidity and mortality rates were above the national norms at this institution.

The sonographer was faced with a legal, moral, and ethical dilemma. The technical supervisor did not want to get involved. The sonographer realized that contact with the higher levels of the hospital's administration, including legal counsel, could bring serious consequences, including dismissal. However, the ethical implications regarding the welfare of the patients compelled the sonographer to arrange a meeting with the chief administrator and the hospital lawyer. After the meeting, the radiologist was told to cease these practices or risk losing his contract to provide services to the hospital. An in-service educational program was held for all obstetricians on staff to review amniocentesis procedures.

This physician was trying to transfer legal liability to the sonographer. Many court cases within the medical field have upheld the legal doctrine of respondeat superior, or the "captain of the ship" doctrine. The presence of the radiologist in the room during the procedure established his supervisory role. The lack of any guidance or response during the procedure does not diminish or transfer the legal responsibility. Including the name of the sonographer in the report does not transfer legal liability. Indeed, because the sonographer is an employee of the hospital, the physician in effect was trying to transfer liability to the hospital. The sonographer must stay within the limits of the institution's job description and national scopes of practice.

BETH ANDERHUB, MEd, RDMS
DIRECTOR, ULTRASOUND PROGRAM
ST. LOUIS COMMUNITY COLLEGE
St. Louis, Missouri

CHAPTER 4

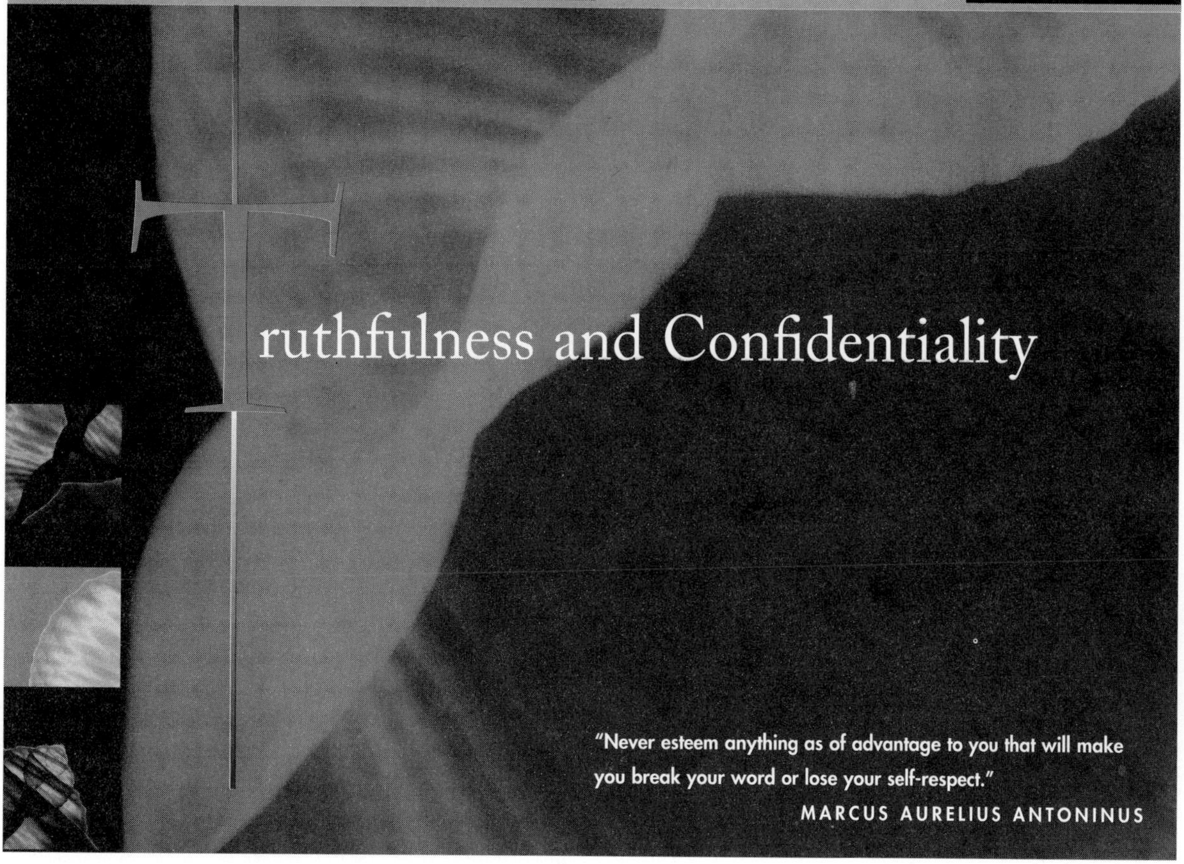

Truthfulness and Confidentiality

"Never esteem anything as of advantage to you that will make you break your word or lose your self-respect."

MARCUS AURELIUS ANTONINUS

LEARNING OBJECTIVES

- Define *truthfulness, veracity,* and *confidentiality.*
- Identify the three variables involved in expectations of truth.
- Recognize circumstances in which a person has a right to the truth.
- List and define three types of obligatory secrets.
- Analyze the importance of the professional secret.
- Cite exceptions to confidentiality.
- Explore and discuss the elements of defamation, including slander and libel per se.
- Recognize situations that may trigger the duty to warn third parties.
- Identify the conflict between confidentiality and disclosure of HIV and AIDS.
- Recognize the statutory obligations regarding AIDS and HIV.
- Define the patient's right of access to medical records.
- Identify ways that the patient's right of access may come into conflict with the ethical and legal principles by which the imaging professional must practice.

CHAPTER OUTLINE

ETHICAL ISSUES

The struggle between confidentiality and truthfulness is a common one in medical imaging, as in all of medicine. Imaging professionals must consider when they must tell the whole truth and in what situations the truth is the same as the whole truth. On the other hand, some truths must be kept confidential. The difficulty for the imaging professional is in knowing what may be ethically concealed and what must be revealed.

Chapter 3 discussed the information required during the informed consent process. This chapter discusses issues regarding truthfulness and confidentiality in imaging professionals' dealings with patients, surrogates, and other health care professionals. For example, should an imaging professional indicate to a patient that she has a spot on her lung and may have a problem if he overhears a physician telling the patient not to worry, the chest x-ray film looks fine, but the patient should have another x-ray film in 6 months?

The chapter also discusses the principles covering situations in which the truth should be kept confidential. For example, must an ultrasonographer conceal from a mother that her 13-year-old daughter is pregnant and desires an abortion?

IMAGING SCENARIO

Several accident victims arrived at the emergency department, and the trauma imaging specialist assigned to perform portable x-ray examinations became involved in a family's fight for life. The mother was critically injured and a strong possibility existed that she might not survive. Her husband was making good progress. The physician told him his wife was dying. The man then insisted that his wife and children be told, but the doctor decided not to tell the wife or children because it would only cause them more pain. The wife died the next day.

The trauma imaging specialist was aware of this interaction because he was busy with chest imaging when the husband requested that his wife be told about her condition. The imaging professional knew this doctor had a history of determining patients' needs, often contrary to their wishes. During one of the imaging procedures, the man asked the imaging professional about what he thought about the doctor, but the trauma imaging specialist declined to share any information with the husband.

Discussion questions

- Should he have explained the doctor's previous style of paternalism to the patient?
- Did the physician have an obligation to tell the patient that she was dying?
- Did the physician have a right to tell the husband about the wife's condition even when she was competent and had no need for a surrogate?
- Should the children have had the right to know that their mother was dying?

TRUTHFULNESS/VERACITY

Definitions

TRUTHFULNESS
Truthfulness is conformity with fact or reality.

VERACITY
Veracity is the obligation to tell the truth and not to lie or deceive others.

Truthfulness is defined as conformance with fact or reality. However, because the perception of fact and reality may change, truthfulness is a somewhat fluid concept. *Veracity* is defined as the obligation to tell the truth and not to lie or deceive others. Veracity and truthfulness have long been regarded as fundamental to the establishment of trust among individuals, and they have a special significance in medical imaging and other health care relationships. Imaging professionals and patients may have differing perceptions of veracity and truthfulness. Imaging professionals may believe in telling the whole truth, no matter how painful, but the patient's need to know the truth may be entirely different.

Circumstances for Expectations of the Truth

Truthfulness is summed up in two commands: "Do not lie and you must communicate with those who have a right to the truth."[1] The first command leaves the imaging professional free to not communicate to avoid telling a lie, and the second constrains the professional to share information only with those who have a right to the truth.

LIE
A lie is a falsehood told to another who has a reasonable expectation of the truth.

PLACE OF COMMUNICATION
The place of communication is the environment of the expectation of truth.

ROLE OF COMMUNICATION
The role of communication is the relationship between the communicators, which may have an impact on the expectation of truth.

A lie is a falsehood told to a person who has a reasonable expectation of the truth.[1] The ethics of lying is judged in terms of consequences for the individual and society. The expectation of truth varies with the following conditions:

1. Place of communication
2. Roles of the communicators
3. Nature of the truth involved

All three of these conditions are related to the obligation of confidentiality and the right to privacy (Figure 4-1).

If an imaging student asks a clinical instructor about pathology on an image within earshot of a patient, he or she does not have a reasonable expectation of truth. The question asked in this place of communication may force the instructor to avoid telling the truth about the pathology if the patient might overhear the conversation and become distressed. However, students do have an expectation of truth if they ask the same question in the classroom during a film analysis class. This is an example of expectations varying with the place of communication.

If an imaging student asks the clinical coordinator for information about another student's performance on a clinical competency examination, the inquiring student has no reasonable expectation of truth because of the role of the two communicators. The score of another student is not the student's concern, and the clinical coordinator has an obligation of confidentiality to all the students.

The nature of the truth involved alters the expectation of truth in questions concerning private matters. If an imaging professional asks a student or any other person about finances, sex life, or anything of a personal or private nature, the imaging professional should not expect a truthful answer.

Overly curious imaging professionals may be found in many imaging departments, just as overly curious people are found in every profession. Such people have

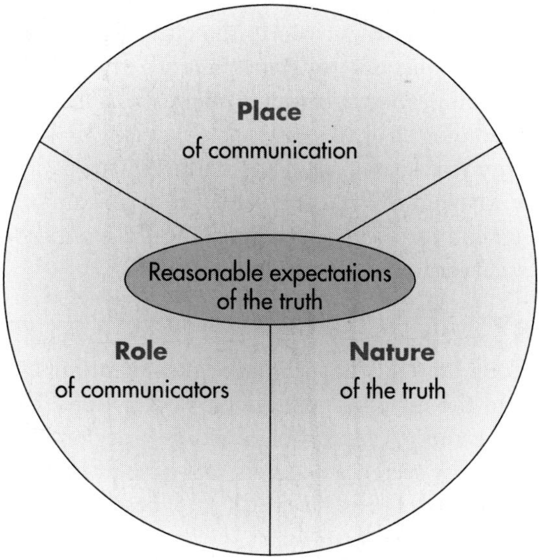

FIGURE 4-1
Components of a reasonable expectation of truth.

unreasonable expectations of the truth. The temptation is to tell these people to mind their own business, but this is not always the wisest course in the hospital setting, where teamwork is imperative. "Snoopy" imaging professionals have no reasonable expectation of the truth and need to be counseled about their unprofessional behavior.

However, concealment of the truth is not necessarily a lie, and in certain situations the imaging professional does not have to tell the whole truth. Thus the question arises concerning the circumstances in which people have a right to the truth.

RIGHT TO THE TRUTH

A person has the right to truthful communication during the informed consent process, when making decisions about treatment, and when making important nonmedical decisions. If a patient's computed axial tomography (CAT) scan reveals that lung cancer has spread to the liver and other vital organs, the patient needs to be informed of this terminal condition to make necessary plans. If the information is not provided, the patient may not make necessary arrangements or deal with family, psychologic, and spiritual issues. In cases of terminal illness, such practical needs often are more important than medical needs to the patient.

In the previous section the patient's expectation of the truth was mentioned. This is an important consideration for the imaging professional because the patient may ask about the outcome of an imaging examination fully expecting the truth. However, the truth about the examination may entail information only a radiologist or the patient's physician can provide. Therefore the imaging professional in this situation cannot provide the whole truth to the patient. For example, if the patient expects the truth to be an answer to the question "Has my cancer spread?", the imaging professional must deal with the patient's expectation of truth by being considerate, understanding, and explaining to the patient that this information will be provided by the radiologist or the patient's physician. Imaging professionals do not have the authority to discuss pathologic findings with patients. In this type of dilemma, they have to avoid the whole truth even if they are certain that the cancer has spread. Image interpretation for the patient is the purview of the physician, who is qualified to answer follow-up questions as well.

CONFIDENTIALITY

CONFIDENTIALITY
Confidentiality is the duty owed by health care providers to protect the privacy of patient information.

SECRET
A secret is knowledge a person has a right or obligation to conceal.

Considerations of confidentiality are as important as truthfulness in the discussion of patients' rights and the imaging professional's obligations. Confidentiality concerns the keeping of secrets: "A secret is knowledge a person has a right or obligation to conceal. Obligatory secrets are secrets that arise from the fact that harm will follow if a particular knowledge is revealed. . . . These are the natural secret, the promised secret, and the professional secret."[1]

OBLIGATORY SECRETS (BOX 4-1)

Natural Secrets

Information shared in a natural secret is by its nature harmful if revealed. An imaging professional may know that a patient has acquired immunodeficiency syndrome (AIDS) but has the obligation to keep the knowledge confidential. If the information were made public, the person positive for human immunodeficiency virus (HIV) could have difficulties gaining employment and might be persecuted socially. However, some situations are more complex. For example, a cardiovascular technologist is involved in a procedure that indicates a patient is in need of immediate cardiac surgery, but the patient decides not to have the surgery. Within a few days the technologist boards an airplane and realizes the pilot is the patient who determined not to have cardiac surgery. Should the technologist tell the airline or some other authority of the pilot's medical condition? Does the harm that may come from concealing the natural secret outweigh the harm to the former patient?

BOX 4-1 OBLIGATORY SECRETS

An obligatory secret is a confidence that will result in harm if it is revealed. Obligatory secrets have three types:

1. Natural—A secret that by its nature would be harmful if revealed
2. Promised—A secret the receiver has promised to conceal
3. Professional—A secret maintained to protect the patient, society, and profession

Promised Secrets

Knowledge a person has promised to conceal is a promised secret. The harmful effects of breaking a promise complicate professional relationships and discourage the sharing of privileged information that may be vital to patient care. Imaging professionals who cannot be trusted to keep secrets about patients or co-workers not only breach confidentiality, but also lose trust as employees or friends. Proportionality must govern the imaging professional's decisions regarding the divulging of promised secrets. If the risk of keeping the secret outweighs the harm to the patient or friend, the imaging professional must make a decision. For example, if a student technologist knows another student has hepatitis (and has sworn not to tell because graduation is in 1 month and the student with hepatitis has already missed the maximal sick time) and they are both scheduled to scrub for an invasive vascular procedure, the student may choose to confide in an instructor if concerned about the spread of infection, regardless of whether the risk is great. The student's peace of mind is important when it may influence the successful completion of the procedure. The student making such a promise to a classmate may need to reevaluate the ethical implications of such a promised secret.

Professional Secrets

The most binding of the obligatory secrets is the professional secret. When professional secrets are revealed, both the patient and the imaging profession are harmed. This damage to the reputation of the imaging profession harms the community, which depends on a limited number of professionals for imaging services. If people lack faith in imaging professionals, they may choose not to have necessary imaging procedures performed. This in turn complicates the diagnostic process and endangers the health of patients.

The importance of professional secrecy has been recognized by society. A body of laws encourages privileged communication and the maintenance of confidentiality between health care providers and patients. The Patient's Bill of Rights of the American Hospital Association (AHA) describes the importance of professional secrecy in the hospital setting based on the nature of the knowledge, the implied promise of secrecy, and the good of society and the profession (see pp. 11-12).

EXCEPTIONS TO CONFIDENTIALITY

Some exceptions to confidentiality are mandated by state law. They include mechanisms for the reporting of certain types of wounds, communicable diseases, automobile accidents, abuse, birth defects, drug addiction, and industrial accidents. State requirements may differ.

The AHA's Committee on Biomedical Ethics notes the following conditions in which confidentiality may be breached[2]:

> Also subject to state law, confidentiality may be overridden when the life or safety of the patient is endangered such as when knowledgeable intervention can prevent threatened suicide or self-injury. In addition, the moral obligation to prevent substantial and foreseeable harm to an innocent third party usually is greater than the moral obligation to protect confidentiality.

BOX 4-2 EXCEPTIONS TO CONFIDENTIALITY

Wounds	Addictions
Abuse	Family's need to know
Communicable diseases	Public's need to know
Accidents	Third-party payers
Birth defects	

In many jurisdictions, imaging professionals are required to report suspected cases of child and adult abuse. Such situations may involve families with whom they are familiar. They may be urged by the family not to intercede because the abuser is in treatment and the reporting mechanism might deter continued treatment. This may be a difficult situation for the technologist; however, employers expect loyalty to the institution, which includes the reporting of abuse.

Exceptions to confidentiality may be debated in discussions of the family's need to know (as in the case at the beginning of this chapter), exceptions concerning children and adolescents (e.g., abortive processes, treatment for sexually transmitted diseases), medical condition of public figures (e.g., whether Americans have the right to know if the president is in critical condition), use of hospital records for research and billing purposes, and third-party payers (e.g., need for payment balanced against patient confidentiality). Exceptions to confidentiality are further discussed in the legal section of this chapter (Box 4-2).

CONFIDENTIALITY AND AIDS

Imaging professionals usually are not placed in situations in which they must inform patients they have HIV. However, occasionally patients will ask imaging professionals if they are HIV-positive. Imaging professionals must decide based on institutional rules and professional experience whether this information is necessary for the patient to give informed consent. Other situations may be just as difficult. An imaging professional may need to report a fellow technologist who has AIDS and does not take necessary protective measures with patients. Although the revelation may cause grief and loss of social contacts or even employment, the technologist must consider the good of patients and the profession.

Some professionals are deontologists and believe that stricter rules of right and wrong should be used in keeping information confidential. They believe that the act of keeping information confidential is more morally important than the consequences this act may cause.

Because of these differing and often conflicting viewpoints, questions concerning AIDS will continue to be fuel for public debate. However, hopefully a cure or vaccine will be discovered, and the problem will no longer haunt the public and health care professionals.

LEGAL ISSUES

Although ethical dilemmas often arise regarding friction between truth, confidentiality, and secrecy, the law provides some parameters regarding patient confidentiality. One of the most important obligations owed by a health care provider to a patient is the protection of confidences revealed by the patient. As with all duties under the law, however, situations exist in which this duty is not absolute and at times the law imposes a duty to disclose confidential information.

Generally, exceptions to patient confidentiality may be separated into four categories:

1. Patient consent
2. Statutory disclosure
3. Duty to warn third parties
4. AIDS confidentiality and reporting

The law regarding patient consent to release of information, statutory disclosure, and the duty to warn third parties is fairly settled; thus the parameters are fairly clear. However, because of the special characteristics of AIDS and the AIDS epidemic, AIDS confidentiality and reporting present unique challenges to health care workers. A conflict often arises between the general duty to keep confidences and the specific obligation to disclose medical information as part of the duty to warn others. This is complicated by the fear of AIDS, the ignorance about the ways in which it is spread, and the history of prejudice and discrimination against gay men (among whom AIDS is most common). Additionally, a significant rise in HIV and AIDS among heterosexual adults is occurring. Disastrous consequences associated with employment, insurability, and social stigma are threatening for all those affected.[3]

The states have adopted a variety of legislative and administrative approaches to confidentiality and disclosure of information regarding HIV-positivity, AIDS-related complex (ARC), and AIDS status.[3] This chapter relays information about the state of the law generally; however, imaging professionals may want to speak to legal counsel at their facilities to determine the law in their jurisdictions.

Another area of concern in patient confidentiality is patient access to medical records. The status of patients' rights to their own records has changed over the past decade, and many jurisdictions have enacted statutes allowing patients access to their medical records. This is discussed later in this chapter.

The intentional tort of defamation also results from a violation of confidentiality. Defamation is the uttering or publishing of an unprivileged false statement that hurts another's reputation. Although defamation is generally thought of in the context of a supermarket tabloid, the opportunity may arise in the delivery of patient care and therefore is discussed in this chapter.

BREACH OF CONFIDENTIALITY

Confidentiality is the duty owed by health care providers to protect the privacy of patient information. This duty stems largely from the right to privacy, but courts have imposed liability based on statutes defining expected conduct, ethical duties owed to the patient,[4] breach of the fiduciary duty to maintain confidentiality, and breach of contract or implied contract between patient and physician or health care facility.[5]

Regardless of the origin of the duty of confidentiality, imaging professionals clearly have an obligation to keep medical and personal information about patients in confidence. As health care providers, imaging professionals have access to a vast amount of information on patients. Breach of the duty to hold information in confidence may cause liability for the individual and the facility.

In certain circumstances, remedies are available through state and federal statutes to compensate patients for breach of confidentiality. Case law has confirmed that courts do award compensation for these breaches of confidence.[6]

The Code of Federal Regulation and many state laws provide a high level of confidentiality for patients receiving drug or alcohol abuse treatment.[7] These requirements have generally caused providers to refuse to disclose even whether a certain individual is a patient. Many states have enacted legislation protecting confidential information regarding HIV or AIDS status, and courts have been willing to allow claims based on these statutes. Unless disclosure is mandated by patient consent, statute, a duty to warn third parties, or the special circumstances surrounding HIV and AIDS, imaging professionals have a clear duty to maintain confidentiality of medical and related information regarding patients.

DEFAMATION

DEFAMATION
Defamation is the making of a false statement to a third party that is harmful to another's reputation. In the medical imaging setting, defamation may occur if something false that is harmful to one's reputation is said to another about a patient, a patient's family member, a visitor, another employee, or a physician.

The tort of defamation is based on the right to maintain a good reputation.[8] As stated earlier, the opportunity for defamation may arise in the delivery of patient care and is therefore worthy of discussion.

Defamation is the uttering or publishing of an unprivileged false statement that hurts another's reputation. If the publication is oral, the defamation is slander; if written, it is libel. The publisher must be at fault at least to the degree of negligence. Harm must have resulted from the publication of the false and defamatory statement. Because the statement must be false, the truth is a total defense to defamation. However, a jury trial may be necessary to determine the truth.

Additionally, if the false statement concerns criminal activity; a loathsome disease such as AIDS or venereal disease; business, trade, or professional misdeeds; or unchastity, no specific injury need be proven. These situations are termed *slander per se* or *libel per se.* Because no injury must be proven in libel or slander per se, the only facts to be proven are that a false and defamatory statement or writing was made to another person and the teller or writer was at least negligent in telling it.[8]

DISCLOSURE OF CONFIDENTIAL INFORMATION

Third parties seek access to records for many reasons. New health care providers may require a patient's previous medical history. Insurance companies may require patient records for billing purposes. Law enforcement agencies may seek to examine medical records for a variety of reasons, and attorneys often require them to investigate disability, personal injury, and medical malpractice claims. Life, health, disability, and liability insurers use medical records for insurability determination and claim processing; employers and credit investigators also may seek to review patient medical records.[3] These disclosures are greatly important to patients

IMAGING SCENARIO

You are an imaging professional who has heard a rumor that a family practice physician, Dr. Smith, whose office is in your clinic, is being investigated for Medicare fraud. You happen to be chatting later with your friends at the monthly get-together of your old imaging technology school classmates and share the rumor you heard. One of your classmates is married to a family practice physician just finishing his residency. Although you were not aware of this, apparently Dr. Smith had been negotiating with your classmate's husband to join his practice. Because of the rumor you retold, he decides not to join Dr. Smith's practice, nor is Dr. Smith able to recruit any of the other finishing residents. Interestingly, you later find out the rumor was false.

Discussion questions

- Are you liable for defamation?
- Is it libel or slander?
- Is it per se?
- Does Dr. Smith have to prove he was damaged?

because risk of loss or denial of employment, insurability, and credit may be at stake and they may be embarrassed by revelations in the medical records.[3]

Patient Consent

Patients may explicitly consent to the release of medical information in their records. Presumed consent exists when access is granted to treating providers, when a patient is transferred from one provider to another, and when emergency treatment requires access to records.[3] Patients have been found to have waived their rights to confidentiality when they put their mental or physical state at issue in a lawsuit. In the case of a lawsuit, a subpoena (a request signed by a judicial officer requesting records when a lawsuit is in progress) may be issued. The subpoena must specify the records to be disclosed.

Patient consent for in-house use of medical information (e.g., in-house quality assurance committees, Joint Commission on Accreditation of Health Care Organizations [JCAHO] inspections, state institutional licensure reviewers) is implied from the patient's agreement to treatment, although some states have statutes expressly authorizing access.[3]

Release of patient information to outside reviewers is governed by state law with the exception of Veterans Administration (VA) hospitals and other federal facilities. Some statutes allow state boards to review patient records to evaluate provider misconduct, and the Medicare program requires providers to allow peer review organizations access to records of Medicare patients. In the absence of statutory or judicial support for release of information to outside reviewers, the sharing of information from patient medical records poses liability risks.

Third-party payers are the most common outside requesters of medical information. Patient consent is necessary for this release; however, most insurers require patients to authorize release of information when they file claims for payment.[3] Some states have enacted statutes for disclosure to insurers without authorization to determine responsibility for payment.

Statutory Disclosure

State public health laws require medical professionals and institutions to report a variety of medical conditions and incidents, including venereal disease; contagious diseases such as tuberculosis; wounds inflicted by violence; poisonings; industrial accidents; abortions; drug abuse; and abuse of children, elderly people, and people with disabilities. The justification for overriding patient confidentiality is the state's interest in protecting public health.[3]

STATUTORY DUTY TO REPORT
The statutory duty to report is the legal obligation to report a variety of medical conditions and incidents, including venereal disease; contagious diseases such as tuberculosis; wounds inflicted by violence; poisonings; industrial accidents; abortions; drug abuse; and abuse of children, elderly people, and people with disabilities.

The statutory duty to report certain medical conditions or incidents may extend to the imaging professional. Because laws vary from state to state, imaging professionals should seek advice from legal counsel at their institutions regarding conditions or incidents that must be statutorily reported.

Duty to Warn Third Parties

The duty to maintain confidentiality may come into conflict with the duty to disclose information to third parties to warn them of a risk of violence, contagious disease, or some other risk. Generally, the duty to warn is based on statute (such as the venereal disease or child abuse reporting statute) and the duty established through case law to warn identifiable third parties threatened by patients. In recent years, the most difficult conflict between confidentiality and duty to warn has arisen in cases in which AIDS or HIV information is involved; this dilemma is discussed in its own section.

DUTY TO WARN THIRD PARTIES
The duty to warn third parties is the obligation to disclose information to warn third parties of a risk of violence, contagious disease, or some other risk.

Case law imposes a duty to warn third parties regarding psychiatric dangerousness. The precedent-setting case was *Tarasoff v Regents of the University of California*[9] (Box 4-3). The duty to warn in *Tarasoff* involved a specific, identifiable third party. Unfortunately, the duty to warn is not clear cut in case law. Some courts have limited it to cases in which the endangered party is readily identifiable, and some have rejected the duty to warn entirely.[3] Other jurisdictions have expanded the duty to include readily identifiable individuals who would be at risk of the patient's violence or even whole classes foreseeably at risk. Some cases attempt to identify third parties who must be warned, typically in situations of psychiatric dangerousness.[3]

Situations involving the duty to warn of psychiatric dangerousness are not routine to the imaging profession. However, because this duty extends to all medical professions, imaging professionals may want to seek clarification on the extent of the duty imposed in their jurisdictions, particularly if their facilities have a psychiatric or mental health component. Patients sometimes feel very comfortable with imaging professionals and volunteer information they have not shared with their physicians, psychiatrists, or therapists. This situation is more likely to arise when the imaging procedure takes an extended amount of time and the imaging professional and patient are alone in the room throughout the procedure, such as during many nuclear medicine studies.

Duties to disclose confidential information regarding contagious diseases have been imposed on physicians. Foreseeable third parties and parties at risk who must be

BOX 4-3 CASE STUDY IN DUTY TO WARN THIRD PARTIES

Tarasoff v Regents of the University of California involved an outpatient (Posenjit Poddar) who was under the care of a psychologist (Dr. Moore) at the Cowell Memorial Hospital of the University of California. During the course of treatment, Dr. Moore learned from Poddar that he intended to kill Titiana Tarasoff because she had spurned Poddar's romantic advances.

On the basis of this information, Dr. Moore had the campus police detain Poddar, apparently at the hospital. Poddar was released shortly afterward. Despite disagreement among the psychiatrists, the final decision was that no further action should be taken to confine Poddar. This judgment proved to be mistaken; 2 months later Poddar shot and then repeatedly stabbed Tarasoff.

The plaintiffs, Tarasoff's parents, brought a wrongful death claim against the four psychiatrists. The plaintiffs claimed that the defendants should be liable because they failed to confine Poddar and because they failed to warn Tarasoff or her parents about Poddar's threat. Liability was not found for failure to confine Poddar, but it was found for failure to warn the identifiable third person in danger.

warned in these situations have been held to include family members, neighbors, and anyone who is physically intimate with the patient. Generally, the standard for the imposition of liability is whether reasonable care was used.[3] This means that if a court were to find that a reasonable person would have found a duty to warn a particular third person, but the physician failed to warn, liability would be found. This duty extends to other health care professionals. However, situations in which an imaging professional would be required to disclose such information are rare. In reality, this issue would likely arise only in an atmosphere in which an imaging professional was working in a clinic or physician's office also as a medical assistant. In such a situation, the imaging professional should become aware of the policies and procedures of the office or clinic regarding disclosure, ensuring that the duty to warn third parties is addressed. Generally, if accurate disclosure of information is made in good faith for a legitimate purpose, courts are reluctant to impose liability for that disclosure.[10]

AIDS Confidentiality and Reporting

The unique challenge to health care professionals presented by the special characteristics of AIDS and the AIDS epidemic arises from the ever-present conflict between the general duty to keep confidences and the specific obligation to disclose medical information as part of the duty to warn others. Because of the fear of AIDS, the ignorance about the ways in which it is spread, the history of prejudice and discrimination against gay men (among whom AIDS is most common), and the disastrous consequences associated with employment, insurability, and social stigma, many argue that the strictest confidentiality regarding information about a patient's HIV status is essential.[3]

The proponents of confidentiality state that any risk of disclosure discourages persons who may possibly be HIV-infected or have AIDS or ARC from seeking

IMAGING SCENARIO

A nuclear medicine technologist is performing a bone scan on a patient from the inpatient mental health center. Extra images are needed, and consequently the patient is in the imaging room for almost an hour, alone with the technologist for most of that time. The patient obviously wants to talk and starts telling the technologist about his brother-in-law, who the patient feels is responsible for his involuntary committal into the facility. The patient gets increasingly upset and eventually tells the technologist about a plan to get even with the brother-in-law when he is released. The plan involves tampering with the brakes on the brother-in-law's car, which the patient assures the technologist he can do because he was formerly a mechanic.

Discussion questions

- Does the technologist have a duty to ensure the brother-in-law is warned?
- Is the fact that disclosing this information will likely have an effect on the patient's continued hospitalization and treatment a consideration in this situation?
- Does a duty to disclose outweigh the basic duty to keep patient confidences?
- What should the technologist do if a statute mandates strict confidentiality regarding mental health treatment?

testing and counseling; in this way, they argue, the duty to warn undermines the possible success of voluntary AIDS testing programs. Moreover, because the HIV virus cannot be spread through casual contact, unlike many other contagious diseases, proponents of confidentiality feel the risk posed by not informing family members and partners of the possibility of infection does not outweigh the damage done to the patient by the violation of confidentiality. They argue that the rate of infection through heterosexual genital intercourse is very low (about 0.1% per exposure) and therefore no duty to warn heterosexual partners should be implemented, because casual heterosexual partners are unlikely to become infected.[3]

The argument in favor of warning is that longer-term partners may not have yet been infected and so should be warned. The possibility of transmission to unborn children may justify warning infected women who may potentially bear children.[3] Current statistics indicate that in 80% of all cases, transmission of HIV from an infected mother to the child can be prevented. However, successful prevention of transmission requires the mother's knowledge of her infection and subsequent prenatal testing.[11] Despite recent strides in treatment techniques, the strongest argument for warning is that at present AIDS is incurable and therefore prevention is essential.[3]

The conflict is evident. Strict confidentiality may encourage persons who may be infected to come forward to be tested and voluntarily modify their behavior to avoid infecting others, but limited disclosure may better protect persons who may be exposed to possible infection (Box 4-4).

BOX 4-4 CURRENT EVENTS IN AIDS CONFIDENTIALITY AND REPORTING

Proponents of AIDS and HIV disclosure may have received an unfortunate but very real boost to their arguments. On October 28, 1997, while awaiting sentencing on drug charges, twenty-year-old Nushawn Williams faced accusations that he knowingly infected at least nine women and girls with the AIDS virus in rural upstate New York.

Chataqua County Health officials said they had documented at least nine HIV cases in which Williams is suspected of infecting sex partners as young as 13. Health officials stated that at least half of the women were infected after Williams learned he had HIV about a year ago. Williams gave New York City health officials 50 to 75 names of women he claimed he'd had sex with, according to New York State Health Commissioner Dr. Barbara DeBuono.

Discussion question

- Does this current event change your attitude toward disclosure of medical information? Why or why not? In what way does it affect your attitudes about truthfulness and confidentiality?

From: *The Boston Globe,* October 28, 1997.

Legislation

The states have adopted a variety of legislative and administrative approaches to confidentiality and disclosure of information regarding HIV-positivity, ARC, and AIDS status.[3] This section provides information about the general state of the law; however, imaging professionals may want to speak to legal counsel at their facilities to determine the status of the law in their jurisdictions.

Most states have adopted statutes mandating strict confidentiality of AIDS-related information. However, the range of exceptions to these confidentiality requirements is quite broad. All states require physicians to report AIDS cases to state public health authorities, and a number of states also require reporting of cases of asymptomatic HIV infections, usually anonymously. Other states have adopted laws permitting disclosure of HIV test results to persons at risk of HIV infection from sexual or needle-sharing contacts with the infected person. In these states, physicians are protected from liability whether they disclose or choose not to disclose the information.[3]

In some states, health care workers have a statutory obligation to counsel HIV-infected patients to take special precautions to avoid infecting others and tell their sexual or needle-sharing partners to seek counseling and treatment.[3] If patients indicate that they will not do so, the health care worker's obligation to warn others is defined by the particular state. Some states permit public health authorities to engage in contact tracing or partner notification with respect to AIDS and HIV.

Imaging professionals usually deal only with the strict confidentiality portion of the disclosure laws. However, imaging professionals working in clinics or physicians' offices and also acting as medical assistants may have opportunities to deal with the exceptions to the duty of confidentiality. Imaging professionals who find themselves in such situations should seek the advice of legal counsel to understand the law in their areas.

Another way that AIDS disclosure laws affect imaging professionals as well as hospitals and other health care facilities is in decisions concerning whether to warn patients about HIV-infected staff. Although little evidence exists that HIV is readily transmitted from provider to patient, some courts have found that a duty to warn patients about HIV- or AIDS-infected staff members overrides state and federal confidentiality rules. These cases usually involve surgical situations; some courts have concluded that although the risk of transmission from provider to patient is very low, the risk involves extended uncertainty for a patient exposed to a surgical accident involving a surgeon with AIDS. One case encouraged a special informed consent policy for treatment by HIV-positive providers and policies to limit HIV-positive workers from patient care situations in which they might pose risks to patients.[3]

Again, imaging professionals should be aware of the law in their areas. Although the information in this section may be used as a guide, situations may arise for which the imaging professional can find no easy answers. For example, what should an imaging professional do if she sees a fellow imaging professional she knows is HIV-positive scrubbing in on a cardiac catheterization? This dilemma may be easier to handle if the facility has a policy to prevent HIV-infected staff members from putting themselves in higher patient risk situations (e.g., surgery, invasive procedures). These policies, however, open an avenue of possible liability regarding discrimination in the workplace. Discrimination against people with HIV and AIDS is discussed in Chapter 8.

What if the imaging professional who is HIV-positive is seriously dating a student technologist and indicates to another imaging professional that he has no intention of telling her of his HIV status because he is sure she would not consent to having sexual intercourse? The confidant professional is no longer in a patient-provider relationship, but does she have any duties toward this student? Should she encourage the imaging professional to seek counseling to understand the potential risk to which he is exposing the student? If the HIV-positive imaging professional refuses to seek counseling, does the confidant imaging professional have a duty to discuss the risks and the possible obligation to disclose his status to a potential sexual partner? If the HIV-positive imaging professional is persistent in his decision not to share this information, does the confidant imaging professional have a duty to tell the student?

PATIENT ACCESS TO RECORDS

Medical records have traditionally been viewed by courts as the property of the institutions or practitioners that create and maintain them.[3] However, some courts have recognized a limited property right of the patient to the information in the record.

IMAGING SCENARIO

Mary Smith, a local dentist, had a radionuclide ventriculogram this morning. You, as the nuclear medicine technologist performing the examination, had access to the chart and noticed that this patient was HIV-positive. You used universal precautions, and the examination was performed without event. At lunch in the cafeteria, you tell your nurse friend who works in the emergency department that Mary Smith is HIV-positive. This is overheard not only in the cafeteria but also in the emergency department as your friend tells several of her co-workers. When Mary Smith returns to her practice, she finds that many of her scheduled patients have canceled their appointments. She tracks down the cause of some of the cancellations to information regarding her HIV status, which was discovered from various hospital employees.

Discussion questions

- Do you realize that you breached patient confidentiality by telling Mary Smith's HIV status to your friend?
- Have you also exposed your facility to liability?
- What are possible origins of the duty to maintain this confidence?

Patients' rights of access to their medical records have gained ground over the past decade. Half of the states have now enacted legislation permitting patients access to their medical records, compared with only seven states in 1978.[3] The AHA and the American Medical Association (AMA) have developed policies in favor of patients' rights of access to their own records. Courts may rely on these policies to establish a common-law right of access.[3]

Although progress has been made in allowing patients access to their records, some state statutes still contain many exceptions to the right of access, including provisions that records are accessible only after discharge, only a summary of the records must be given, or the patient must show good cause before access is granted. Opponents of patients' access to their records argue that patients will not understand the information in the records and may become upset and engage in harmful self-treatment. Additionally, they claim it discourages physician frankness and imposes greater administrative costs.[3]

Proponents of access argue that greater access encourages better understanding of and compliance with treatment and improved patient-physician relations and continuity of care. Additionally, they note that patients must know the contents of their medical records before they are able to give truly informed authorization of their release to others.[3] The prevailing view is that patients are helped rather than harmed by access.

Imaging professionals should follow departmental policies and procedures regarding the showing of records and reports to patients. If questions still exist, the medical records department or legal counsel should be knowledgeable regarding the status of the law in the jurisdiction. Generally, however, the best option is to arrange for the interpreting physician to speak to the patient. Imaging professionals who show patients their x-ray films face an additional dilemma because the patients generally ask questions about them and they will either have to not answer at all, answer evasively, or defer to the interpreting physician at that point. If the interpreting physician is not willing to speak to the patient, the imaging professional should assist that patient in finding information by directing the patient to the ordering physician. Imaging departments should have established policies in place on ways to deal with this very common patient request.

SUMMARY

Imaging professionals are expected to tell the truth in situations in which others have a reasonable expectation of the truth. The location of the communication, the roles the communicators have in relationship to one another, and the nature of the material to be communicated are determining factors in the expectation of truth. Contract relationships and special needs are factors that determine whether a person has a right to information.

Of all the types of obligatory secrets—natural, promised, and professional—professional secrecy is the most important because of the damages incurred as a result of its violation. In certain instances, professional secrets may be shared. This occurs most often when the good to be gained by sharing the information outweighs the evil of violating confidentiality, when the law indicates they must be shared, or when special relationships indicate a need for an exception.

The imaging professional has a clear duty to maintain patient confidentiality. However, a small number of exceptions to this duty exist and require the professional to disclose confidential information. Unless a situation meets one of the exceptions to the duty of confidentiality, disclosure may create liability for the individual and the facility.

Common exceptions to the duty to confidentiality include the following:

- Situations in which the patient has consented to the sharing of information
- Statutory disclosures
- Duty to warn third parties
- AIDS confidentiality and reporting

The tort of defamation is another issue of concern with regard to confidentiality. It occurs when a false statement is made to another that harms a person's reputation. Oral defamatory statements constitute slander and written defamatory statements constitute libel. Defamatory statements regarding criminal activity; loathsome diseases; business, trade, or professional misdeeds; and unchastity constitute slander or libel per se; in these situations, no specific injury need be proven.

Truth is a total defense to defamation, although after it is alleged, a trial may be necessary to determine the truth. Defamation in the health care setting may occur when false statements are made about patients, visitors, family members, other employees, or physicians.

The law varies across jurisdictions but is fairly clear on exceptions regarding patient consent, statutory disclosures, and the duty to warn third parties. The law concerning AIDS confidentiality and reporting is not as clear cut as the other exceptions to confidentiality.

Although most states have statutes mandating strict confidentiality, exceptions are numerous and vary from state to state. Imaging professionals generally are not exposed to many situations involving the exceptions to the strict confidentiality duty regarding patient HIV or AIDS status. However, imaging professionals also acting as medical assistants may find themselves involved in dilemmas regarding the duty to disclose and should discover the status of the law in their areas. In addition, imaging professionals may find themselves involved in situations regarding whether to warn patients regarding HIV-infected staff members. They should ask about the status of the law in their state and know the policy in their facility.

Patients' right of access to their own records has gained significant ground in the past decade. However, access is not granted in all states and imaging professionals should know the status of the law in their particular areas. The policy for release of images and reports from the radiology department should be in accordance with state law and the policies of the health care facility. The medical records department is generally a good source of information and is generally willing to provide assistance to ensure the appropriateness of the radiology release policy. If answers are not satisfactorily obtained from the medical records department, legal counsel should be consulted.

One patient access dilemma frequently faced by imaging professionals occurs when patients want to see their x-ray films or other images. Although showing patients their films may not violate the law or professional ethical obligations, answering questions about patient films may put imaging professionals in situations in which they cross the line into interpretation and lead to questions regarding treatment that they cannot answer. Imaging departments should establish policies to deal with this common situation, preferably by referring patients to the interpreting or ordering physician.

ENDNOTES

1. Garrett TM, Baillie HW, Garrett RM: *Healthcare ethics, principles and problems,* ed 2, Englewood Cliffs, NJ, 1993, Prentice Hall.
2. Committee on Biomedical Ethics, American Hospital Association: Chicago, 1985, Author.
3. Furrow B et al: *Health law,* St. Paul, Minn., 1995, West.
4. *Humphers v First Interstate Bank of Oregon,* 696 P.2d 527, 1985.
5. *Doe v Roe,* 400 N.Y. Supp. 2d 668, 1977.
6. *Doe v Roe,* No. 0369 N.Y. App. Div. 4th Jud. Dept., May 28, 1993.
7. Code of Federal Regulation, Title 42, Part 2 (1985).
8. Prosser W, Wade J, Schwartz V: *Cases and materials on torts,* ed 8, Westbury, NY, 1988, Foundation Press.
9. *Tarasoff v Regents of the University of California,* 551 P.2d 334 (Cal. 1976).
10. *Klipa v Board of Education,* 460 A.2d 601 (Md. Spec. App. 1983).
11. American Medical Association: *Policy compendium,* H-20.931, Chicago, 1997, Author.

REVIEW QUESTIONS

1 Define *truthfulness.*

2 Expectations of truth vary with which three conditions?
   a. ______________
   b. ______________
   c. ______________

3 The right to the truth is determined by the ____________ ____________ of the patient in many nonmedical situations (such as in preparing for death).

4 Informed consent and the need to make treatment decisions are examples of conditions for the ______________ ______ ______ __________ .

5 ______________ is concerned with the keeping of secrets.

6 List the three types of obligatory secrets:
   a. ______________
   b. ______________
   c. ______________

7 The most binding obligatory secret is the ______________.

8 Describe the most common exceptions to confidentiality.

9 According to the AMA Committee on Biomedical Ethics, duties to disclose patient information exist in which situations?

10 Which of the following are origins of the duty of confidentiality?
   a. Right to privacy
   b. Statutes
   c. Ethical obligations
   d. Breach of contract issues
   e. All of the above

11 **True or False** The imaging professional must always tell the whole truth.

12 **True or False** The imaging professional has an obligation to the patient, profession, and society to maintain confidentiality.

13 **True or False** Although the duty of patient confidentiality is clear, courts do not allow compensation for breach of confidentiality.

14 **True or False** Imaging professionals owe an absolute duty of patient confidentiality.

15 **True or False** Truth is a total defense against allegations of defamation.

16 **True or False** Defamatory comments regarding a person's AIDS status are slander per se, and damages would not have to be proven.

17 **True or False** Confidentiality of drug and alcohol abuse treatment information is mandated by the federal government.

18 **True or False** Virtually all requests by third parties for records come from new health care providers.

19 **True or False** Imaging professionals do not have to worry about statutory reporting because this duty lies only with physicians.

20 **True or False** The duty to warn third parties extends to the imaging professional.

21 **True or False** Imaging professionals, even if working in clinics and fulfilling the roles of medical assistants, never have to deal with warning people at risk for contagious diseases.

22 **True or False** The existence of legislation mandating strict confidentiality regarding information about patient AIDS, HIV, and ARC status means that disclosure is never appropriate.

23 **True or False** Because the risk of transmission from provider to patient is low, courts have never imposed a duty to warn patients about HIV-infected staff members.

24 **True or False** The risk of patient exposure to HIV increases if the infected staff member is a member of a surgical team.

25 **True or False** Patients always have an absolute right to their records.

26 **True or False** Imaging professionals should feel free to show patients their films and answer questions about them.

CRITICAL THINKING QUESTIONS & ACTIVITIES

1 What is the difference between not telling the whole truth and telling a lie? Why might one be admissible?

2 Cite a situation in which the place of communication is inappropriate for an expectation of truth in medical imaging.

3 Discuss the differences and similarities between natural and promised secrets.

4 If you were HIV-positive, do you think your patients or employer would have the right to know? Why or why not?

5 Should a parent have the right to know a child's physical condition if it involves treatment? Why or why not?

6 Define *confidentiality.*

7 Identify exceptions to the duty to confidentiality.

8 Consider the following situation: With the health care system changing and third-party payers becoming stricter about coverage, imaging professionals (as are all other people) are concerned with their own health care services. Do you think your third-party payer has a right to know your health history and present conditions if they involve a communicable disease or drug history? Should you be able to expect privileged communication between you and your physician? Justify your answers. A group discussion may follow in which each person lists the consequences of the decision and possible alternatives.

9 Discuss situations that may potentially involve defamatory statements about fellow employees or patients.

10 Discuss the devastation a negligent breach of confidence may cause, such as in the scenario involving the dentist, Mary Smith.

Continued

CRITICAL THINKING QUESTIONS & ACTIVITIES—cont'd

11 Does the facility you are affiliated with have a policy regarding HIV-infected workers? If it does not, should it? Is protection of the patient more important than the rights of HIV-infected staff members?

12 Discuss the situation of the HIV-infected imaging professional who intends to put a student at risk through unprotected sexual intercourse. Does the other imaging professional's duty to warn fall under the law or is it only an ethical obligation?

13 Play out a scenario in which a patient wants to see her x-ray films, an imaging professional who believes patients should have a right to access shows her the films, and the patient starts demanding that the imaging professional answer questions regarding the outcome of the study, what it means, and possible treatments. Discuss a better way to handle the situation and play the scenario again.

PROFESSIONAL PROFILE

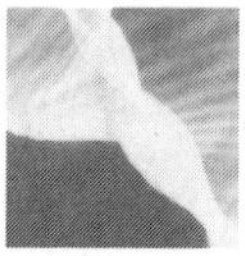

I RECALL my first experience with death and dying as a student radiologic technologist. The image is still quite clear although it happened more than 25 years ago. The department was closed and I got called in from home around 2:30 AM. A second-year student and a staff technologist had also been called.

We wheeled the stretcher with a young man who appeared to be about my age from the emergency department to the radiology department. He had been in a motor vehicle accident and had the gear shift lever from his car sticking out of his chest. We moved him onto the table and began taking films. His breathing became erratic and the staff technologist called the emergency room staff. Soon the entire room was filled with people and equipment. This scene was frantic, with everyone working to try to keep this young man alive. Unfortunately, they were unsuccessful and he died on the x-ray table.

After all the paperwork was completed and the appropriate procedures followed, he had to be moved from the x-ray table to the morgue cart. Because only three radiology personnel were present, we had to help the night supervisor with the actual transporting of the body. I will never forget the way that young man's body felt. It was cold and hard, almost like stone.

That night was the first time I experienced death. That night was the first time I really thought about death. That young man had been alive when we started the examination. He was warm, he had feelings, aspirations, hopes, dreams, and fears. Then he was cold and hard. I thought about what he had experienced. Was he afraid, was he angry, did he see his short life flashing before his eyes? Was it just his body that was dead and did his soul live on to go to heaven or hell as I was taught in grade school, or is this life all there is? This experience bothered me for a very long time. I would wake up in the middle of the night and think of the way this young man's body felt. I would dwell on whether he knew he was going to die, whether he was prepared, what exactly did it mean to die?

I now realize that each person must form his or her own answers to these questions. I also believe that some guidance on the ethical and legal issues of death and dying for the imaging student is appropriate. I was not prepared to deal with these issues as a first-year student and wish that I had been.

CHAPTER 5

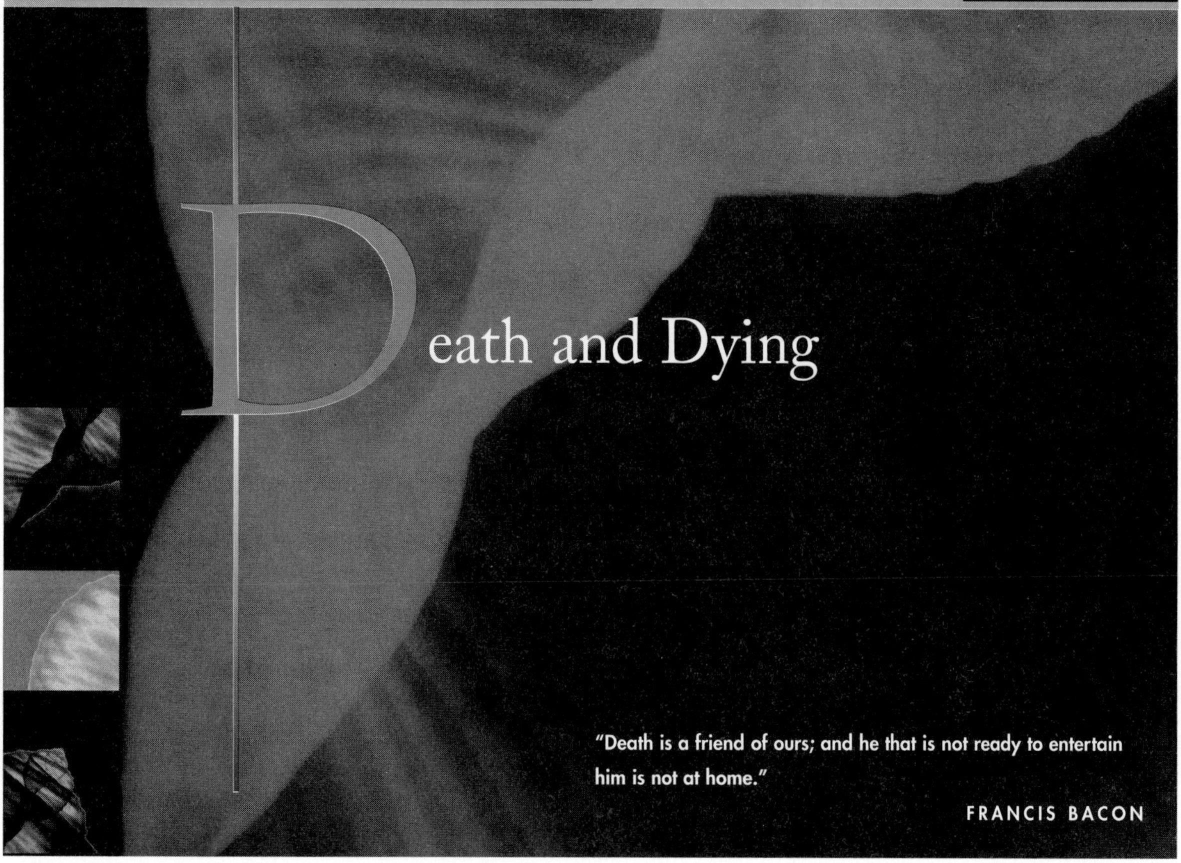

Death and Dying

> "Death is a friend of ours; and he that is not ready to entertain him is not at home."
>
> FRANCIS BACON

LEARNING OBJECTIVES

- Provide definitions of life and death.
- Recognize the differences between the patient's and the imaging professional's role in death and dying.
- Identify the physical and ethical differences between active and passive suicide.
- Evaluate a perceived need for euthanasia.
- Develop arguments for and against the right to die.
- Explore reasons for ethics committees.
- Understand the basis for the patient's right to forego life-sustaining treatment.
- Define *life-sustaining treatment* and its exclusions.
- Identify the difference between living wills and durable powers of attorney.
- Identify the limitations of living wills.
- Define the advantages of durable powers of attorney.
- Discuss the ways in which powers of attorney influence the decision-making process of ancillary people such as physicians, ministers, and specified family members and friends.
- Explore differences in the treatment of persons who have never been competent and competent persons who have become incompetent.

CHAPTER OUTLINE

ETHICAL ISSUES

Imaging professionals often have contact with patients with critical or terminal conditions. Most of the imaging modalities (except radiation therapy) do not involve lengthy contact with patients. Nevertheless, regardless of the length of the therapeutic relationship, the imaging professional will encounter death and dying.

To help the imaging professional deal with questions regarding patients' rights, refusal of treatment, and quality of life, this portion of Chapter 5 discusses ethical concerns surrounding death and dying. The ethical dilemmas of patients and imaging professionals are emphasized.

THE VALUE OF LIFE

Before imaging professionals consider questions of death and dying, they should understand the ethical issues surrounding life. Life may be considered as an element of human autonomy through which a person experiences a sense of self. It is defined as the entire state of the living thing; it encompasses the value of the self

LIFE
Life is the entire state of the living thing.

IMAGING SCENARIO

The portable and trauma team imaging professionals were called to the morgue to perform a radiographic examination on a young man with a gunshot wound. The bullet entered the right temple and was lodged in the brain. The images corroborated forensics that indicated suicide. Before the fatal wound the young man appeared to have been muscular, handsome, and healthy. The youngest imaging professional questioned why such a young man who had his whole life to look forward to would choose such a tragic ending.

The next day another staff imaging professional noted that the young man had recently been diagnosed with an incurable and inoperable brain tumor. This information led to a discussion about the choices people make when they know they will die, perhaps painfully. Did this man have the right to end his life? In what way did the suicide affect his family and friends? Did his situation excuse his suicide? In what ways were the family dealing with not being able to say their final good-byes?

The young trauma imaging specialist wondered what she would do in such a situation. Would she choose to die a slow, painful death or end her life quickly? Did she have the right to determine the quality of her life and choose suicide or euthanasia even if both were illegal or considered immoral by many? How would she respond to a healthy young patient faced with the prospect of an early and painful death? Was there an obligation to counsel about possible treatments and pain-control modalities that was not met or could have been handled better? What impact do these questions have on the professional's compassion and quality of care toward patients?

and is a determining factor in a person's "preconscious" standard of judgment. Thought, analysis, and action come from this fundamental sense of the value of life.

Traditional religious and secular beliefs celebrate the uniqueness of life, but when life begins and the way it ends remain points of contention. The imaging professional should consider the following aspects of life when making determinations in ethical dilemmas[1]:

- Life is the foundation of all a patient's other values.
- Life is the foundation of a patient's rights.
- The preservation and maintenance of a good quality of life are the goals of the patient entering the health care environment.
- A patient is motivated to enter the health care environment when capabilities and potentialities are radically affected. If a patient can regain these capabilities and potentialities, quality of life is greatly improved.
- A patient, except in the most extreme circumstances, has no rational desire greater than the desire for life. Nevertheless, in extreme circumstances a desire for death may not be irrational.

DEFINITIONS OF DEATH

Most people and cultures agree that physical life is a cyclic event with a beginning and an end. The life cycle is generally considered a good to be held in awe and respected. Some believe that the goodness of life may be judged by the decisions a person makes regarding actions and responses to others and the environment. Others believe decisions concerning the goodness of life should be the person's own determination. Many arguments and problems are inherent in this philosophy; they are discussed later in this chapter, as are legal definitions of death, persistent vegetative state, and coma.

THE PATIENT

A discussion of the ethical dilemmas faced by the imaging professional requires a consideration of the ethics of the patient, including questions concerning passive and active suicide. Empathy with the patient provides the imaging professional with insight into these questions.

SANCTITY OF HUMAN LIFE

The ethics of the taking of human life becomes a consideration in a number of patient care situations, and imaging professionals may have to address this issue during their interactions with patients. Respect for the sanctity of human life entails an obligation not to infringe on an individual's decisions regarding life and an obligation not to take human life.[2] Nevertheless, questions about the sanctity of life arise in situations of assisted suicide and when patients are suffering from life-threatening disease or illness.

SANCTITY OF HUMAN LIFE
Sanctity of human life is the ideal underpinning the obligation not to take human life.

SUICIDE

Suicide is the act of knowingly ending one's own life. It may be accomplished either actively or by omitting treatment, which is a passive form of suicide. The individual also must have the intention to die.

SUICIDE
Suicide is the act of knowingly ending one's life.

Several arguments may be made against suicide (Box 5-1). It may be unacceptable for religious reasons—God has loaned life to the individual, and therefore that life is not the individual's to end. Others believe that human life is the greatest of goods and consider it precious. However, what if the patient has tremendous pain and therapy has caused such nausea and weakness that the patient cannot move from bed? Is life "good" at this level of pain and loss of dignity? Harm to the community is another argument against suicide. If one suicide leads to another (as has been observed with teenage suicides), does this not harm the community? Another argument against suicide is the harm it inflicts on family and friends. Suicide denies them time with their loved ones to plan, share, make amends, and say good-bye.

All these arguments have some logic, and laws to control and discourage suicide are based on such arguments. If suicide were declared legal, would more untimely deaths be associated with emotional problems and not just physical problems? Would the broken heart be cured more often with a bullet than with therapy and understanding?

Passive Suicide

Ethically, patients have the right to refuse treatment even if it brings about death. Of course, not all refusal of treatment leads to death. However, would a situation in which a patient knows the refusal of treatment will bring about death much more rapidly be considered a form of passive suicide? Some may consider passive suicide ethical if the good of the act outweighs the bad of the suffering. The following scenario explores some of these issues.

PASSIVE SUICIDE
Passive suicide is the refusal of treatment by a person who knows that refusal will lead to death.

BOX 5-1 ARGUMENTS AGAINST SUICIDE

Many religions forbid it.
Life is the greatest good.
It causes harm to the community.
It causes harm to friends and family.

IMAGING SCENARIO

Two patients are diagnosed with pancreatic cancer, and the computed tomography (CT) scan indicates the cancer has invaded many other organs. One patient has elected to discontinue nourishment to hurry death; the other patient elects to continue all treatment to sustain his life as long as possible. How do personal values, as discussed in Chapter 1, influence the weighing of reasons for refusing treatment as compared with continuing it?

Active Suicide

ACTIVE SUICIDE
Active suicide is the taking of one's own life through a conscious act.

Some people can accept the idea of passive suicide because refusing treatment is a person's right and refusal of treatment does not seem to be an act of violence toward the self. However, when the young man in the imaging scenario on p. 101 shot himself to end his life quickly rather than die a painful and slow death, would some consider this active suicide wrong? Those who oppose suicide do so for various reasons. Some believe that life is sacred and must be cherished. Others believe that only God or some supreme being gives life and only that being should decide when it should end.

Suicide proponents also have their rationale. Many believe suicide is an individual right, analogous to a woman's right to an abortion. If a woman has the right to choose what will happen to her body, shouldn't an individual have the right to choose life or death? Some also argue that it is not only the supreme being that gives us life, that technology also allows humanity to produce life, and if humanity can produce life, why shouldn't it be allowed to decide when it should end? The technology that has been developed to prolong life also is used as an argument against the "God brought life, God should take it away" theory.

THE IMAGING PROFESSIONAL AND SUICIDE

Many imaging professionals have encountered patients who have no hope of becoming well and whose pain can no longer be controlled with drugs. Their lives are full of pain and suffering, and their desire to end their lives may be reasonable. If these patients discontinue treatment, they will suffer but die sooner. They also could overdose and end their suffering quickly. Whether the suicide is active or passive, imaging professionals should be careful not to make judgments. What should be the response of an imaging professional asked to interact with a patient determined to commit passive suicide (Box 5-2)? In what way should an imaging professional approached by a patient who wishes to end life either actively or passively respond? These may be rare situations for imaging specialists, but they must be considered because of imaging professionals' changing interactions with patients and their families. Imaging professionals must recognize that each case is different. They may be required to participate in procedures involving patients who have elected to end nourishment and hydration. The imaging professional must remember that it is the value system of the patient that is important in such situations, not the value system of the imaging professional.

BOX 5-2 REASONS FOR THE IMAGING PROFESSIONAL'S DUTY NOT TO COOPERATE WITH ACTIVE SUICIDE

1. Assisting in or supplying the means to suicide is generally illegal.
2. Health care providers are devoted to healing.
3. Assisting in suicide is incompatible with professional obligation.

EUTHANASIA

Suicide is taken one step further when another person becomes involved. Euthanasia is the act of painlessly putting to death a person suffering from an incurable and painful disease or condition. Physician participation in euthanasia, or assisted suicide, has stirred much controversy recently (Box 5-3). The legal issues surrounding physician-assisted suicide are discussed in the legal section of this chapter.

EUTHANASIA
Euthanasia is deliberately ending the life of another to end suffering.

ACTIVE EUTHANASIA
Active euthanasia is the ending of another person's life by an aggressive method to end suffering.

PASSIVE EUTHANASIA
Passive euthanasia is the ending of another person's life by withdrawing treatment.

Euthanasia may be either passive or active. The difference between the two lies in the methods, not the consequences. Passive euthanasia may be committed through the withholding of nourishment or through a decision not to perform cardiopulmonary resuscitation (CPR) on a patient who has stopped breathing. It is considered legal in certain instances because no one delivers a method of death. "Nothing" is done and that "nothing" leads to death. Active euthanasia is the performance of a specific act on the request or behalf of the patient to end life.

Professionals in the medical imaging services may see patients with terminal diseases, patients in horrible pain, or those in a persistent vegetative state (PVS) (The medicolegal definition of PVS is discussed in the legal section of the chapter.) These imaging professionals may struggle with whether they should perform procedures that will add to the patient's pain and loss of dignity and autonomy (e.g., barium enemas). They may imagine themselves in the patient's position and hope

BOX 5-3 PHYSICIAN-ASSISTED SUICIDE

The physician who has drawn the most attention to the current controversy over physician-assisted suicide is Dr. Jack Kevorkian. Dr. Kevorkian is a pathologist by training, although he has not held a position on a hospital staff since 1982.

In 1989, inspired by a patient who was quadriplegic and wished for someone to turn off his respirator so that he could end his life, Dr. Kevorkian began to invent a suicide machine to enable disabled people to kill themselves by merely touching a button. A 54- year-old patient with Alzheimer's disease was the first person Kevorkian assisted to commit suicide in 1990.

Dr. Kevorkian acknowledges having been present at more than 50 deaths since 1990. He has been arrested several times for performing doctor-assisted suicide, and charged, tried, and acquitted of murder.

Dr. Kevorkian's actions have provoked a furious debate over the rights of terminally ill patients to choose suicide and whether physicians can ethically be involved in patient suicide. Many United States physicians believe that assisting in suicide violates their Hippocratic oath, the promise to prolong and protect life. Others have argued that assisting in suicide actually upholds the oath, the promise to relieve the suffering of patients who are in pain and have no hope of recovery.

The Clarke College for the Interdisclipinary Study of Contemporary Issues: *Assisted suicide in context,* Carlisle, Penn., 1997, Dickenson College.
CNN Interactive: *Jack Kevorkian, assisted-suicide advocate,* Atlanta, Ga., 1997, Cable News Network.

that someone who cares about them would help hasten their death. At the same time, they should consider the consequences for the person "helping" them. The imaging professional should also remember that they should not base their decisions on their own personal values. The patient's values and needs are the important issues in these decisions.

The legal ramifications of euthanasia, especially active euthanasia, are tied to the act of murder. Indeed, many people believe that they are the same, and this is the basis for euthanasia being generally illegal in the United States. In Holland, where euthanasia has become an accepted procedure, some health care professionals and ethicists wonder whether this acceptance will become a slippery slope leading to the overuse and misuse of euthanasia. For example, will the euthanasia of a patient suffering from acquired immunodeficiency syndrome (AIDS) lead to the deaths of unwanted types of individuals and ethnic cleansing? No policies are currently in place regarding who makes these decisions, and the ways in which controls should be established remain controversial.

SLIPPERY SLOPE
A slippery slope is present when one act leads to another and then to another at an accelerating rate.

Morally and legally, the questions involving passive euthanasia are more complex. The passive withdrawal of nourishment from a patient in a PVS seems less awful than the active euthanasia of a patient who is conscious and aware. However, after health care professionals and family members start making judgments for handicapped neonates or patients who are incompetent, in a PVS, old, or senile, the implications for patient autonomy become serious. Who decides who is fit to live ? Does a person have to have consciousness and decision-making ability to be worthy of life? The potential for development and quality of life must be considered. If a neonate has a chance to develop and live (not necessarily by traditional standards), should that chance be given? Should cost and distribution of resources issues play a role in such decisions?

DEVELOPMENT
Development is the ability to grow and continue the life process.

The controversies surrounding the euthanasia of neonates often are related to the issues in the abortion debate. Questions regarding when the fetus has a right to life, self-determination, and dignity have yet to be resolved. When aborting a fetus that can wave its arms and legs and suck its thumb is legal, but the legality of letting an anencephalic neonate be an organ donor is still in question, do such perceptions confuse the issues surrounding the processes of life and death? Ultrasonographers required to participate in fetal ultrasound examinations that may lead to abortive procedures must learn to deal with these dilemmas based on professional standards and personal conscience.

ABORTION
Abortion is the expulsion or removal of a usually nonviable fetus (a fetus that cannot live outside the uterus at that time).

Euthanasia of patients at the beginning of life raises serious ethical questions. So too does the active or passive euthanasia of elderly people. Elderly patients should be evaluated by imaging professionals as individuals with value, not as "old people" who have lived long lives and are somehow expendable. The intellectual capacity and strength of elderly people may be failing (although many elderly people retain a high degree of intellectual capability), but a human being does not have to be a perfect specimen to have a reason for living. The fear of pain and loss associated with death may be as great to an 85-year-old as it is to a 35-year-old. The age of the patient should never interfere with the imaging professional granting the best care possible.

PATIENTS' RIGHTS REGARDING EUTHANASIA

The ethical questions surrounding the possibility of a patient having a right to active euthanasia are complex. Consider the patient in hospice care with pain control who has been diagnosed with invasive liver and pancreatic cancer by a CT scan and has undergone radiation therapy for pain. Does this patient have the right to self-determination and a "good death" through euthanasia if all of these procedures have not lessened the pain, or must the patient continue to be in pain?

The exercise of rights requires a self; proponents of patient-chosen euthanasia consider it an act of self-determination. Therefore the person seeking euthanasia must completely understand the nature and consequences of the request. The person must be competent and as informed as possible. Ideally the person should have experienced the five stages of coming to terms with death:

1. Denial
2. Anger
3. Bargaining
4. Depression
5. Acceptance

In a scenario of legalized euthanasia, only after going through these phases would the patient be considered ready to make the decision regarding the commission of euthanasia.

ADVANCE DIRECTIVES AND SURROGATES

Advance directives and surrogates (who act on behalf of patients and may make decisions and grant consent for them in quality-of-life judgments) are increasingly important elements in decisions regarding euthanasia. Written explanations of patient wishes in the form of living wills or advance directives hasten the processes leading to passive euthanasia. However, active euthanasia is still generally illegal, and many roadblocks stand in the way of its becoming an accepted procedure. The idea of lethal injections evokes perceptions of "doctors of death" and "angels of mercy." This is not the life-giving image most health care providers wish for themselves. Even with an advance directive, a patient in a PVS or a burn patient in hideous pain would have great difficulty finding a health care professional willing to run the risks inherent in active euthanasia. This is why active euthanasia currently is generally performed by a loved one—someone willing to run the risk of murder charges and a prison cell.

SURROGATE
A surrogate is a person who substitutes for another, often in decision-making processes.

Proponents of active euthanasia feel society has more compassion for animals that are in pain and suffering than it does for suffering human beings. Those opposed to active euthanasia believe the improved methods of pain control can enhance the quality of a patient's life. A concern for patient rights and autonomy may require imaging professionals to consider these divergent interpretations of the ethics of euthanasia.

Imaging professionals are charged with working to provide for the good of the patient's health; many feel this entails an obligation to maintain life under any circumstance. However, the patient's autonomy and freedom to choose treatment options may come into conflict with this ethical and professional obligation. In some instances imaging professionals may need to help prepare patients for death and help themselves and their patients to see that death is not always an enemy.

QUALITY OF LIFE

QUALITY OF LIFE
Quality of life encompasses essential traits that make life worth living.

Quality of life has different meanings for different people. Factors influencing quality of life may include the capability of performing normal biologic functions, the stability of the powers of intellect and creativity, and emotional contact with others. Some persons may demand a maximum of these factors to feel their lives are worth living, whereas others have minimal needs and find the simplest interactions to be the rewards of life (Figure 5-1).

Most people fall into the middle of the quality-of-life spectrum. They may not demand maximal health and happiness, but they do not want to live in agonizing pain and without hope. The use of living wills is one way to ensure that people's wishes regarding treatment in relation to their quality of life are honored. Living wills identify specific treatments to be initiated or discontinued when patients become terminally ill, are in great pain, or find themselves in a life-threatening situation. If a living will is not present and the patient's wishes are not known, quality-of-life decisions are difficult to make. In such situations, the minimal requirements for quality of life must be recognized. Imaging professionals must not pass judgment on others facing these dilemmas; they can only be decided for the individual by the individual—not by others.

ETHICS COMMITTEES/SERVICES FOR PATIENTS WITH TERMINAL ILLNESSES

Many hospitals have formed ethics committees to help health care professionals address the ethical problems surrounding termination of treatment and related issues. These committees have several missions. First, they educate the hospital, its employees, and its other constituencies. Second, they develop policies regarding problem areas, especially the problems of death and dying. Third, they act as advisory consultants to health care providers and families.

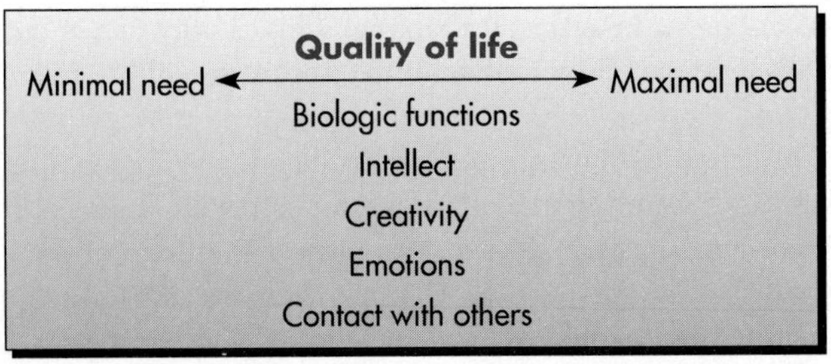

FIGURE 5-1
Factors involved in quality-of-life decisions.

Ethics committees serve in an advisory capacity only. Ideally, their recommendations are exercised with practical wisdom in the patient's best interest.

In addition to ethics committees, other services exist in the health care community to provide aid to terminally ill patients. Included are hospice care, home health care services, mental health services, social services, organizations for persons with specific terminal diseases, pastoral and religious services, and others. Often these services provide support to terminally ill patients and their families and help deal with the many issues involved in the final portion of the life cycle.

THE FAMILY IN DEATH AND DYING

Medical imaging personnel often interact with patients' families during the dying process[3]:

> At a certain point in the dying process, the family members become secondary patients in need of information about the state of affairs and emotional support. Too often the families are neglected and left to fend for themselves. Yet, insofar as the health care professionals are dedicated to relieving suffering, the duty of compassion is in the role of all care givers. The duty to relieve suffering demands concern for the well and the living as well as for the ill and dying. Families, as well as those who are patients in a legal sense, have needs that should be respected.

Imaging professionals must interact with families in a manner that exhibits a caring and professional attitude. They must be approachable and ready to comfort grieving family members, no matter how difficult this duty may be. Professional empathy is crucial for the well-being of the patient and the patient's family.

LEGAL ISSUES

Many aspects concerning the patient's right to die remain unresolved. In fact, the only well-resolved issue is the recognition of the common-law right to choose the form of treatment. As was stated in previous discussions of battery and informed consent, Justice Cordozo established in the 1914 *Schloendoff* case that "every human being of adult years and sound mind has a right to determine what shall be done with his own body." This finding also underpinned the right to forego treatment—because patients have a right to determine whether to consent to a particular treatment, they also have a right to refuse to consent to a particular treatment.[4a]

The principle that competent patients have a right to forego life-sustaining treatment was not articulated by any court until 1984.[5] According to that finding, the competence of the patient is crucial to whether he or she has a right to forego life-sustaining treatment; the method by which that right is exercised also is relevant. Unfortunately, courts have been reluctant to give a formal definition of competence. This section discusses legal and medical definitions of death and persistent vegetative state, competence, guidelines for its determination, and its significance for the right to die and the vehicles used to further that right.

As previously noted, laws vary by jurisdiction, and judicial decisions from one jurisdiction are not binding in others, although they may be considered by the deciding court.

DEFINITIONS OF DEATH

The Heart-Lung Definition of Death

For centuries, death has been evidenced by the contemporaneous cessation of heart and lung function. These functions were related to such a degree that the cessation of breathing would lead almost immediately to the cessation of heart function and the cessation of heart function would lead almost immediately to the cessation of breathing. Additionally, the cessation of these functions was accompanied or immediately followed by cessation of all cognitive activity, all other brain function, and all responsiveness generally.

Because the disappearance of any heartbeat and the cessation of breathing were the simplest to identify, and because the advent of the stethoscope made the determination of heartbeat easier, the heart and lung test of death became not only the evidence of death but also the actual definition of death. Today, all states accept this heart-lung definition of death as at least an alternative definition; when a person's heart and lung function has irreversibly ceased, that person is dead. Today, most deaths in the United States are determined by application of the traditional heart-lung definition of death.

Brain Death

New technologic developments demanded a new definition of death. Two such developments were sophisticated ventilators and heart-lung machines. These machines allowed the heart to keep beating and the lungs operating even in the absence of any other indications of life. Before this technology, the heart and lungs could not function without brainstem activity. After this technology, the heart and lungs could continue to function even in the absence of a functioning brainstem.

The advent of successful organ transplantation techniques also rendered the heart-lung definition of death inadequate. Irreversible damage to the brainstem eventually leads to the cessation of function of the heart and lungs. However, this cessation takes some time, time in which potentially transplantable organs might not receive sufficient oxygen. Rather than delay the certain declaration of death and destroy the possibility of transplanting healthy organs, many suggested that death be declared early enough to make the organs available for transplantation.

Ultimately, the heart-lung machine and organ transplantation techniques led to the acceptance of alternative criteria for death—the traditional heart-lung criterion in most cases, and the newer "brain death" criterion in cases in which the use of life-support systems or the potential for use of the decedent's organs for transplant made the traditional criteria impossible or inefficient.

In 1968, the Ad Hoc Committee for the Harvard Medical School to Examine the Definition of Brain Death proposed a new criterion to reflect the need for an alternative definition of death. This committee called the new criterion "irreversible coma," which includes the following characteristics: unreceptiveness and unresponsiveness, no movement or breathing, no reflexes, and a flat electroencephalogram.

The Committee's use of the term *irreversible coma* has caused some problems, because the condition they were describing is not a coma at all, but irreversible lack of function of the entire brain.

Persistent Vegetative State

The term *irreversible coma* is now sometimes used to describe a patient in a PVS, when all higher brain function is lost. PVS differs from brain death because the brainstem continues to function and the body is not dead. Patients in a PVS may even seem to be awake but have no awareness of themselves or their environment. Imaging professionals should always treat these patients with respect and compassion.

DETERMINATION OF DEATH

The Committee also recommended some procedures for the declaration of death: the ventilator should be removed after death is declared; the physician (and not the family) should make the decision to declare death; the physician may choose to consult with others (although the physician may choose not to) before declaring death; and the declaration should not be made by one with an interest in the subsequent use of the tissue of a patient.

The Committee's recommendation led to legislation (first in Kansas) in an attempt to codify this definition. Much controversy ensued, including versions of statutes promulgated by the American Bar Association, the American Medical Association, and several other organizations. Eventually, in 1980, the National Conference of Commissioners on Uniform State Laws promulgated the Uniform Determination of Death Act of 1980 (UDDA),[6a] which has now been adopted in many states. This Act provides that an individual who has sustained either (1) irreversible cessation of circulatory and respiratory functions or (2) irreversible cessation of all functions of the entire brain, including the brainstem, is dead. A determination of death must be made in accordance with acceptable medical standards.

Where no statute for brain death exists, courts have been willing to accept the brain death definition in the unusual cases in which it is an issue, although the courts would clearly prefer the decision be made by legislative action.

Because the declaration of death is a scientific medical matter, it is governed by medical standards, not legal ones. The UDDA provides that this determination is to be made "in accordance with accepted medical standards."[6a] Because those medical standards change over time and depend on the diagnostic tools available in different times and different places, it makes sense for good medical practice to determine what counts as good evidence that the definition of death has been met.

Currently, a physician declaring death based on brain death criteria is constrained by good medical practice to confirm the absence of any response to stimulus and the absence of any spontaneous respiration and cardiac activity. The Ad Hoc Committee's advice that life-support systems not be removed before the declaration of death is made and that any physician involved in the subsequent transplantation of organs from a deceased person not be involved in the declaration of death remain good advice, although not required by law.

Generally, a physician declaring death has a certain leeway regarding the time death is declared. Although delaying declaring death for financial gain (such as an extra day billed to the hospital) is inappropriate, it may be very appropriate to delay declaration of death a few hours so that loved ones may see their family member "alive" once more.

CPR has traditionally been treated differently from other forms of life-sustaining treatment. CPR is the only form of life-sustaining treatment that is provided routinely without the consent of the patient, and it may be the only medical treatment of any kind that is generally initiated without an order of a physician. The following sections discuss orders that further a patient's wishes not to be resuscitated.

DIRECTIVES

In response to a highly publicized case in 1976, many states adopted statutes designed to give formal recognition to some form of written directives by patients; these directives are generally called *living wills.* The case concerned the right to die of Karen Ann Quinlan, a victim of a car accident who was kept alive on a ventilator and with feeding tubes for years, against what Quinlan's family and friends felt was her will.[6] This section discusses the current state of the law regarding living wills and the treatments that can be withheld when a living will exists.

Another well-publicized case helped further the development of the law regarding advance directives and living wills. This was the 1990 case of Nancy Cruzan,[7] in which the Supreme Court in a split decision refused to allow life-sustaining measures to be withdrawn from a woman in a PVS (Box 5-4).

Although the outcome of the Cruzan case was controversial for proponents of the right to die, Justice Sandra Day O'Connor established in her opinion (which concurred in the result with the majority, but differed in the reasoning) some further guidelines and encouragement for use of durable powers of attorney. The durable power of attorney for health care decisions is an advance directive that is not limited to terminal conditions or specified treatments but instead appoints a person or persons to assume a substitute decision-maker role in the event the patient is unable to make decisions. This section discusses the durable power of attorney as an advance directive tool. Moreover, this section discusses situations in which no advance directive is in place.

BOX 5-4 CASE STUDY: NANCY CRUZAN

On the night of January 11, 1983, Nancy Cruzan lost control of her car as she traveled down Elm Road in Jasper County, Missouri. The vehicle overturned, and Cruzan was discovered face down in a ditch without respiratory or cardiac function.

Paramedics were able to restore her breathing and heartbeat at the accident site and she was transported to a hospital in an unconscious state. It was estimated that Cruzan was deprived of oxygen for 12 to 14 minutes. She remained in a coma for approximately 3 weeks and then progressed to an unconscious state. In order to ease feeding and further the recovery, surgeons implanted a gastrostomy feeding and hydration tube in Cruzan with the consent of her then

BOX 5-4 CASE STUDY: NANCY CRUZAN—cont'd

husband. Subsequent rehabilitative efforts proved unavailing. She died in 1990, after lying for years in a Missouri state hospital in what is commonly referred to as a *persistent vegetative state:* generally, a condition in which a person exhibits motor reflexes but evinces no indications of significant cognitive function.

After it became apparent that Nancy Cruzan had virtually no chance of regaining her mental faculties, her parents asked hospital employees to terminate the artificial nutrition and hydration procedures. All agreed that such a removal would cause her death. The employees refused to honor the request without court approval. The parents then sought and received authorization from the state trial court for termination.

The Missouri trial court decided that Nancy had a fundamental right to die based on the communication to a friend that if sick or injured she would not want to continue her life unless it was halfway normal. The Missouri Supreme court reversed by a divided vote and the case ended up in the United States Supreme Court. The Supreme Court refused to allow the life-sustaining measures to be withdrawn. The court felt that clear and convincing evidence did not exist that Nancy Cruzan desired to have artificial hydration and nutrition withdrawn.

Modified from *Cruzan v Director, Missouri Dept. of Health,* 497 U.S. 261, 190, 110 S. Ct. 2841, 2857, 1990; *in re Cruzan* 110 S. Ct. 2841 (1990).

The role of imaging professionals regarding advance directives may appear small. However, nearly every day of imaging practice involves the provision of care for patients with terminal illnesses. An awareness of the state of the law enables imaging professionals to be more sensitive to patients, know the patients' legal rights, and ensure that both patients and professionals realize the options available to direct health care in the future.

TERMINAL ILLNESS
A terminal illness is a condition that leaves the patient irreversibly comatose or will lead to death within a year.

PHYSICIAN-ASSISTED SUICIDE

As stated earlier, physician participation in euthanasia, or assisted suicide, has stirred much controversy recently. The United States Supreme Court decided in June 1997 that states may ban assisted suicide but did not prohibit states from passing laws that would allow physician-assisted suicide. This United States Supreme Court case upheld the state laws in New York and Washington banning physician-assisted suicide. However, the Supreme Court also left the door open for states to allow physician-assisted suicide, if they so desire. The Court found no constitutional right to physician-assisted suicide. The Court also upheld New York's decision that a distinction exists between withholding medical treatment and actively assisting suicide.

The result of this decision by the United States Supreme Court is that each state may decide for itself whether the physicians in its state should be allowed to assist a terminally ill patient who desires to end life by prescribing medication that is intended to do just that. Many states currently have legislation in effect that outlaws physician-assisted suicide. Oregon is the only state at present with a law allowing physician-assisted suicide.

The Oregon voters passed a law in 1994, known as the Oregon Death with Dignity Act, by the narrowest of margins (51% to 49%) in an election with the lowest voter turnout since 1978. The Act allows doctors to prescribe lethal medications to end the lives of patients thought to be terminally ill who desire to end their lives. Shortly after passage, the law's constitutionality was challenged. The voters were asked to decide whether to repeal this law in a special election held November 4, 1997. Although some confusion occurred during this vote (to repeal the law, a YES vote was required in the November election; to keep the law, a NO vote was required), the law was not repealed.

Although technically physician-assisted suicide is legal in Oregon, the U.S. Drug Enforcement Administration (DEA) has said that doctors who prescribe lethal medications to assist a suicide violate the federal narcotics law and could lose their licenses to prescribe drugs. This determination was issued by DEA Administrator Thomas A. Constantine in a letter to Republican Congressman Henry Hyde dated November 5, 1997. It was overturned in June of 1998 by Attorney General Janet Reno.

The debate will no doubt continue. Ethical and social issues are as important as the medical and legal ones. One social fear in the acceptance of physician-assisted suicide is that it could open the door for extension of such a practice to minorities, including physically and mentally disabled and indigent people. Proponents of this argument cite the medical excesses that occurred in Nazi Germany. However, the medical community has a greater interest in the outcome. First, ending a patient's life goes against the words of the Hippocratic oath. Second, many feel this power over life and death puts the physician in the role of God or executioner, depending on personal viewpoint.

Defenders of assisted suicide state that physicians are faced with this dilemma daily and act on it. Proponents of this argument say that a person who is facing certain death has the right to inflict his or her own death to hasten the process and alleviate pain and that physician involvement would make the process easier. The argument also has been made that a physician helping to cause death is no different than one who withholds treatment to allow death to occur. As stated earlier, the Supreme Court has found a difference exists.

Another physicians' concern about legalization of physician-assisted suicide involves the mental status of the patient at the time of the request. Proponents of this argument believe that most terminally ill patients seek suicide not because they are ill, but because they are depressed, and that the depression is treatable. This argument further states that it is not good to circumvent the dying process, which includes the stages of denial, anger, bargaining, depression, and acceptance.

Another argument involves concern that legalizing physician-assisted suicide will lead to a decrease in end-of-life care to patients who do not choose to die. Proponents of this argument draw attention to the Netherlands, where physician-assisted suicide is legal. The argument is that in the Netherlands, palliative care has suffered and hospice care lags behind that of other countries, whereas in the U.S., pain management research and palliative care methods are rapidly improving. These proponents argue that this is evidence that science and compassion can work hand in hand.

Opponents of assisted suicide, including all associations of physicians and hospitals in the United States, argue that the main function of medicine is to heal and not to help die, and that legalization would provoke an alarming increase in the number of suicides. This opinion is reflected in the American Medical Association's position on physician-assisted suicide, as it is stated in AMA Opinion 2.211, which follows[9]:

> Physician assisted suicide occurs when a physician facilitates a patient's death by providing the necessary means and/or information to enable the patient to perform the life-ending act (e.g., the physician provides sleeping pills and information about the lethal dose, while aware that the patient may commit suicide.)
>
> It is understandable, though tragic, that some patients in extreme duress—such as those suffering from a terminal, painful, debilitating illness, may come to decide that death is preferable to life. However, allowing physicians to participate in assisted suicide would cause more harm than good. Physician assisted suicide is fundamentally incompatible with the physician's role as healer, would be difficult or impossible to control, and would pose serious societal risks.
>
> Instead of participating in assisted suicide, physicians must aggressively respond to the needs of patients at the end of life. Patients should not be abandoned once it is determined that cure is impossible. Multidisciplinary interventions should be sought including specialty consultation, hospice care, pastoral support, family counseling, and other modalities. Patients near the end of life must continue to receive emotional support, comfort care, adequate pain control, respect for patient autonomy, and good communication.

COMPETENCE AND LIFE-SUSTAINING TREATMENT

Whether a patient has the right to forego life-sustaining treatment, and the method by which that right can be exercised, depends fundamentally on whether that person is competent to make the decision. Courts have tried to deal with the issue of competence regarding life-sustaining decision making using the traditional law of guardianship and conservatorship. This assumes that a person is either legally competent or incompetent for all legal and medical purposes. More recently, some courts have rejected the all-or-nothing approach and have recognized the concept of "decisional" or "variable" competence. This concept accepts that a person may have the attributes to make particular decisions at some times but not at others. Another presumption that has never been given much credence by the courts is that a person is competent unless a court makes an alternate finding.[10]

COMPETENCE
Competence is the ability to make choices.

In practice, these definitions do not suffice, because strict adherence to these principles makes medical care for the incompetent impossibly burdensome by substantially increasing the caseload of the courts.[10]

Courts have been reluctant to articulate a formula for determining competence. This is true even when the court has had to address specifically the competence of patients to forego life-sustaining treatment.

The most widely accepted test to date to determine patient competence comes from the 1980 President's Commission for the Study of Ethical Problems in

Medicine and Biomedical and Behavioral Research. The Commission found that the capacity to make competent decisions requires, "to a greater or lesser degree," each of the following[10]:

- Possession of a set of values and goals
- The ability to communicate and understand information
- The ability to reason and deliberate about one's choice

Unfortunately, each of these elements is somewhat ambiguous and difficult to apply. Although this test may assist courts in making judicial determinations of competence, it provides little practical help in the determination of whether a patient is capable of making the decision to forego life-sustaining treatment.

Fortunately, tools are available to facilitate efforts by competent people who wish to make medical decisions before they become incompetent. One of these tools is the living will, which generally allows patients to state in advance (in addition to other treatment preferences) that in the event of terminal illness, they wish to forego life-sustaining treatment. Another tool is the durable power of attorney for health care decisions. This directive is broader than a living will and provides for a substitute decision maker to make health care decisions when the patient is not able.

NO-CODE ORDERS

As discussed earlier, CPR has traditionally been treated differently from other forms of life-sustaining treatment. CPR generally is provided unless a formal "do not resuscitate" (DNR) order is entered on the patient's chart.

Historically, CPR was not discussed with patients. The mid-1980s fear of legal ramifications for not performing CPR, even when obviously futile or inconsistent with the wishes of the patient, exacerbated this lack of communication with the patient about CPR. This resulted in "slow codes" or "pencil DNRs," meaning staff members would be instructed to provide resuscitation guaranteed not to be successful (for example, be slow in calling the code). Other institutions used a certain colored removable dot on the patient's chart to indicate a "slow code" should be called. The common thread of these practices was that no record not to resuscitate the patient would be left.

The reaction to this process was the development of formal hospital policies that provided for open and honest decision making on DNR issues. Today, generally accepted principles of medical ethics require that hospitals maintain such policies, and many hospitals have delegated this responsibility to their ethics committees. Today, any hospital without such a policy could face legal liability for its absence should a patient inappropriately be resuscitated or not resuscitated because of the uncertain reaction of a nurse, physician, or health care worker within the institution. Imaging professionals must know the status of each patient they are treating regarding CPR status. This includes knowing where in the patient's medical record to find this information and consistently checking this status.

Legislation requiring specific procedures within the state has followed in only one state, New York. The ensuing statute is very precise and complicated. Health care providers had feared that legislation would ensue for all states, creating a system of medical care governed by a crazy quilt of procedures required by statutes, each a little different from the other, but no other state has followed suit.

LIVING WILLS

The 1976 Karen Quinlan case started a trend of statutes to provide formal recognition to some form of written directive by patients. These "living will statutes" often differ significantly; this situation prompted the Uniform Health Care Decision Act of 1994, which formulated a uniform statute that could be adopted by states. Unfortunately, states have been reluctant to adopt it. One significant variable in state statutes is a definition of who may execute a living will. Some states say only competent adults may enact a living will,[11] others allow living wills to be executed for children by their parents, and yet others do not permit patients with terminal illnesses to enact living wills, apparently out of fear that the illness puts patient competence at risk.[10]

Generally, living wills become effective on signing; however, some states have a waiting period for effectiveness. Under the Uniform Rights of the Terminally Ill Act, a living will becomes effective as soon as it is communicated to the physician of a patient who is both terminally ill and incompetent.[12] In many states and under the Act, the living will is suspended during pregnancy, especially if the fetus might be born alive if life-sustaining treatment is continued.[10] In most states, living wills never expire but may be revoked or changed.[10]

Conditions and Treatments Covered by Living Wills

Living wills generally apply in cases of terminal illness. However, in most living will statutes, terminal illness is variously defined or not defined at all. Under the Uniform Rights of the Terminally Ill Act, the living will applies in cases of terminal conditions, which it defines as incurable or irreversible illness.[10] After the Cruzan decision, some states amended their statutes to include irreversible coma and PVS as well as terminal conditions.

Just as living will statutes do not apply to all conditions, they also do not apply to all treatments. Some statutes specify that patients may choose to forego life-sustaining treatment or maintenance medical care; unfortunately, such terms, if defined at all, usually are defined in ambiguous or circular ways.[10]

About half the states explicitly exclude nutrition and hydration from the treatments that may be withdrawn. The constitutional validity of these exclusions is still controversial, especially after the Cruzan case.[10] The Uniform Rights of the Terminally Ill Act is the broadest form of advance directive statute; it applies to any health care decision.[6]

Process of Executing a Living Will

The formalities of enacting a living will also vary from state to state, although they usually are not as strict as those involved in executing a last will and testament. Usually at least one witness is required; some states exclude health care workers and potential heirs from being witnesses.[10] Unfortunately, such limitations exclude exactly the people who are most likely to talk to patients about such decisions and help them execute the document.

Effect of a Living Will

Statutes vary from state to state, but generally the statutes permit health care workers to carry out patient requests without fear of legal consequences, including civil and criminal liability.[10] Most statutes also assert that taking actions permitted by the document does not constitute suicide for any purpose, and physicians' and others' cooperation in the process does not constitute assisting suicide.[10]

Many statutes require physicians who do not wish to carry out the requests of patients with living wills to transfer them to other health care providers who will.[9] Failure to transfer a patient to a professional who will carry out the wishes expressed in a living will may give rise to professional action in some states, including licensing action against the offending health care worker.[10]

Coercing someone into signing a living will, destroying or hiding a living will, forging another person's living will, failing to record the existence of a living will, or making medical care or health insurance coverage conditional on the existence of a living will may give rise to civil or criminal liability.[10] No cases exist, however, in which a health care professional has been sanctioned for any action taken in accordance with a living will.[10]

DURABLE POWERS OF ATTORNEY FOR HEALTH CARE DECISIONS

A durable power of attorney is a document executed by a competent person (the principal) to appoint another (an agent) to make health care decisions when the principal becomes incompetent. Any competent adult may be appointed as an agent under durable power of attorney statutes. An alternate agent may be appointed if the appointed agent is unable or unwilling to act.

Durable powers of attorney may be limited in time, scope, or method of decision making at the discretion of the principal executing the document. For example, a principal may designate a person to make decisions regarding life-sustaining treatment, decisions that do not involve life-sustaining treatment, or any other subclass of decisions. An agent may be required to consult with designated others before making health care decisions or applying principles articulated in the document.

Agents are expected to apply the principle of substituted judgment when making health care decisions; that is, they are to make the decisions the principal would make if the principal were competent. However, the durable power of attorney document may specify other principles to be used by the agent to make decisions. Virtually no practical limits exist to the restrictions and conditions that may be placed on agents in durable powers of attorney for health care decisions.[10]

Durable power of attorney statutes became popular after the Cruzan decision in 1990. In her separate opinion, Justice O'Connor stated that she approved of durable powers of attorney and commented that the "practical wisdom" of such documents has been recognized by several states.[10] She also suggested that durable powers of attorney, which she described as "valuable additional safeguard[s] of the patient's interest in directing his medical care"[10] might have constitutionally protected status. Her opinion further indicated that courts may find the Constitution requires states to follow the decisions of an appointed surrogate.[10]

The reasons that durable powers of attorney for health care decisions have become accepted so quickly by ethicists, physicians, medical institutions, and the law are easy to understand. They allow patients to decide who shall make health care decisions for them and thus help safeguard autonomy.

Because durable powers of attorney do not require patients to anticipate what treatments are required in the event of incapacitation, they are much less likely to give rise to questions and concerns over whether patients have changed their minds than are living wills. Because it appoints a particular decision maker instead of defining a particular decision, a durable power of attorney allows the decision maker to consult physicians and family members about proposed treatments. Although a durable power of attorney is not inconsistent with a living will (a principal may instruct an agent to follow the wishes expressed in the living will), it is generally a far broader document that may be applied to all health care decisions.

FAMILY CONSENT LAWS

Another concept involved in health care decisions by substitute decision makers has become law in many states. This is the concept that when no advance directive exists, physicians and health care facilities should look to family members to make health care decisions. Some states have adopted statutes to give formal recognition to a practice that is based in common sense and has been accepted for a long time.

These statutes vary from state to state, but generally they become effective only when a patient becomes incompetent; some require a certification of incompetence before the family is authorized to make health care decisions. The statutes authorize designated close family members to act on behalf of the patient, but never in the same hierarchy as is used to determine inheritance of the patient's estate. All these statutes require that a patient's designation (e.g., through a living will or durable power of attorney) be followed so no conflict with the patient's wishes occurs.

These statutes have been the subject of very little litigation. This is probably because all they do is bring formal recognition to an arrangement that is merely common sense and has been in use for a long time.

ABSENCE OF ADVANCE DIRECTIVES

When no advance directive or family consent statutes are applicable to provide for decision making for incompetent patients, courts have attempted to protect the principle of autonomy by allowing others to make health care decisions on behalf of incompetent persons. The decision maker (i.e., a family member, a person appointed by the court, sometimes the court itself) must look at all potentially trustworthy sources of information and determine with sufficient reliability the decision the patient would make if competent.

Courts deciding such cases have used different tests to determine whether treatment may be withdrawn based on the strength and certainty of the articulation of the patient when competent and on the current condition of the patient. In one of the most frequently cited cases on the subject, the Karen Quinlan case, the court ordered that the "clear" and "unequivocal" desire of the patient to terminate treatment be carried out.[13] However, as the New Jersey Supreme Court stated in the *in re Conroy* case, if the desire of the patient is neither clear or unequivocal, any apparent desire for the termination of treatment is honored only if the burdens of continued life clearly outweigh the benefits of treatment.[14] The Conroy court went on to state that if the patient has never made any expression about whether life-sustaining treatment should be continued, such treatment must be continued unless doing so is inhumane.[14]

PATIENTS IN A PERSISTENT VEGETATIVE STATE

Only a short time after the Conroy case articulated the tests to determine whether life-sustaining treatment should be withdrawn, the inappropriateness of these tests for patients in a PVS became apparent. The Jobes court explained PVS by quoting the trial testimony of Dr. Fred Plum, who stated: "[Persistent] vegetative state describes a body which is functioning entirely in terms of its internal controls. It maintains temperature. It maintains heartbeat and pulmonary ventilation. It maintains digestive activity. It maintains reflex activity of muscles and nerves for low level conditioned responses. But there is no behavioral evidence of either self-awareness or awareness of the surroundings in a learned manner."[15]

A person in a PVS has no chance of return to a cognitive state, although the body of a patient with this condition may be maintained, sometimes without use of a ventilator, for years and perhaps decades. The Jobes court pointed out that the criteria used for evaluation of incompetent patients should not be used for patients in a PVS. Instead it said that if the particular patient clearly would have refused treatment under the circumstances, treatment should be withdrawn. If, however, the patient's wishes are not clear, "the right of a patient in an irreversibly vegetative state to determine whether to refuse life sustaining medical treatment may be exercised by the patient's family or close friend."[15] This liberal approach to patients in a PVS has been accepted in theory by many states.[10] As Justice Stevens pointed out in his Cruzan dissent, every court that has heard a request to terminate life-sustaining treatment for a patient in a PVS has ultimately approved the request—except the Cruzan court itself.[16]

PATIENTS WHO HAVE NEVER BEEN COMPETENT

If a patient has never been competent (e.g., if a patient has been profoundly mentally disabled since birth), the substituted judgment standard to determine the kind of life-sustaining treatment the patient would want is difficult to apply. Courts are divided on which standard to apply in such situations.[10] One court stated, "We recognize a general right in all persons to refuse medical treatment in appropriate circumstances. The recognition of that right must extend to the case of an incompetent, as well as a competent patient, because the value of human dignity extends to both."[15] It further asserted that the choice is not to be made by asking what a majority of competent people would choose, but rather by determining with as much accuracy as possible the wants and needs of the individual involved.[17]

Other courts have not been as concerned with the autonomy and dignity of persons who have been disabled since birth and think the "best interest" standard should be applied. The New York Court of Appeals, which has narrowly defined even a competent patient's right to forego treatment, has declared that adults who have been incompetent since birth should be treated the same as children.[18] It also has established a default position requiring treatment in virtually all cases. As the court pointed out, a "parent or guardian has a right to consent to medical treatment on behalf of an infant. The parent, however, may not deprive a child of life sustaining treatment, however well intended."[18]

SUMMARY

The value of life and its impact on the imaging professional's ethical decision-making abilities influence choices concerning death and dying. Suicide, euthanasia, and problems surrounding quality of life are all issues that imaging professionals face in their work.

Some may consider passive suicide ethical if the good of the act outweighs the bad (proportionality). Others may consider active suicide ethical in certain situations for the same reason. Nevertheless, this does not mean that the patient has the legal right to commit suicide; suicide and euthanasia are still illegal in most states.

It is generally illegal for imaging professionals to participate in active euthanasia or a patient's active suicide even if the patient is terminally ill. However, in certain instances they may be involved in passive suicides or euthanasia by not performing procedures on patients who have given orders not to be revived with heroic measures if their hearts fail (no-code orders) or patients for whom nothing else can be done medically.

The patient's right to forego life-sustaining medical treatment stems from the common-law right to choose the form of treatment. The reasoning behind the right to forego life-sustaining treatment is that if patients have the right to determine whether they consent to a particular treatment, they also have the right to refuse to consent to a particular treatment.

This principle was explicitly articulated in a 1984 case stating that competent patients have a right to forego life-sustaining treatment. As suggested by this ruling, the competence of patients is fundamental to whether they have a right to forego life-sustaining treatment and the method by which that right is exercised.

Unfortunately, courts have been reluctant to define competence formally. In fact, definitive tests of competence are virtually impossible to articulate. The issue of the inability of a patient who has become incompetent to choose to forego life-sustaining medical treatment was brought to the attention of the world in 1976 through the Karen Ann Quinlan case. This case led many states to pass living will statutes to give formal recognition to some form of written directives by patients. Although living wills serve a useful purpose, their use is limited to patients with terminal conditions. Moreover, the treatment that may be withheld is limited to life-sustaining care, often specifically excluding nutrition and hydration.

Another well-publicized case, the 1990 Cruzan case, helped further the development of the law regarding advance directives. Although the Missouri Supreme

Court refused to allow the withdrawal of life-sustaining treatment, the opinion written by Justice O'Connor established some guidelines and encouragement for the use of durable powers of attorney.

A durable power of attorney for health care decisions is an advance directive that is not limited to terminal conditions or specified treatments but instead appoints a person or persons to assume a substitute decision-maker role if the patient becomes unable to make decisions. It is a much broader tool than a living will and in general allows health care decisions to reflect more accurately the wishes of the patient.

Although these laws do not appear to have a great impact on them, imaging professionals should be aware of them. Nearly every day of practice in imaging involves the provision of care for patients with terminal illnesses. An awareness of the state of the law enables imaging professionals to be more sensitive to these patients and their wishes and know their legal rights. It also enables them to ensure that both professionals and patients realize the options available to direct their health care in an always uncertain future.

ENDNOTES

1. Husted GL, Husted JH: *Ethical decision making in nursing,* ed 2, St Louis, 1995, Mosby.
2. Garrett TM, Baillie HW, Garrett RM: *Healthcare ethics, principles and problems,* ed 2, Englewood Cliffs, NJ, 1993, Prentice Hall.
3. Beauchamp TL, Perlin S: *Ethical issues in death and dying,* Englewood Cliffs, N.J., 1978, Prentice-Hall.
4. Veatch RM, Fry ST: *Case studies in nursing ethics,* Philadelphia, 1987, J. B. Lippincott.

4a. *Schloendoff v Society of NY Hospitals,* 105 N.E.92 (N.Y. 1914).

5. *Bartling v Superior Court,* 209 Cal. Rptr. 220 (Cal. App. 1984).
6. *In re Quinlan,* 355 A.2d 647 (N.J. 1976).

6a. *Uniform Determination of Death Act,* 12 U.L.A. 340 (Supp. 1991).

7. *Cruzan v Director, Missouri Dept. of Health,* 497 U.S. 261, 190, 110 S.Ct.2841, 2857 (1990).
8. *In re Cruzan,* 110 S. Ct. 2841 (1990).
9. American Medical Association: *Policy compendium,* 1997; *Decisions near the end of life,* 1991; *Physician-assisted suicide,* Dec 1993; updated June 1996.
10. Farrow B et al: *Health law,* St. Paul, Minn., 1995, West.
11. *Iowa Code Annotated,* Section 144A.3(1) (1997).
12. Uniform Rights of the Terminally Ill Act, Section 3, 9B, U.L.A. 118 (Supp. 1993).
13. *In re Quinlan,* 355 A.2d 647(N.J. 1976).
14. *In re Conroy,* 486 A.2d 1209, 1232 (N.J. 1985).
15. *In re Jobes,* 529 A.2d 434, 438 (N.J. 1987).
16. *Cruzan v Director, Missouri Dept of Health,* 497 U.S. 261, 348-49, 110 S.Ct. 2841, 2881, Stevens J, dissenting (1990).
17. *Superintendent of Belchertown State School v Saikewicz,* 370 N.E.2d 417, 427 (Mass. 1977).
18. *In re Storar,* 438 N.Y.S.2d 266, 240 N.E.2d 64 (N.Y. 1981).

REVIEW QUESTIONS

1 Life is the __________ __________ of the living thing.

2 Death is the loss of ____________________ and considered part of the ________________ ________________.

3 List three reasons why suicide may be considered wrong:
   a. ____________________
   b. ____________________
   c. ____________________

4 Define *euthanasia.*

5 In what ways do advance directives and living wills assist the health care provider?

6 Define *persistent vegetative state.*

7 List three factors involved in quality-of-life decisions:
   a. ____________________
   b. ____________________
   c. ____________________

8 What is the difference between active suicide and active euthanasia? When may each situation present itself in medical imaging?

9 Discuss the ways in which patient rights may be interfered with and upheld by the law.

10 In what way may an imaging professional cooperate with passive suicide or passive euthanasia?

11 When may an imaging professional ethically be involved in passive euthanasia?

12 **True or False** Patients have the ethical right to refuse treatment.

13 **True or False** Imaging professionals may assist in active suicide.

14 **True or False** Active euthanasia is not against the law in the United States.

15 **True or False** The right to forego life-sustaining treatment is based on the principle of autonomy.

16 **True or False** The right to forego life-sustaining treatment was first articulated by Justice Cordozo in 1914.

17 **True or False** Courts have articulated definite rules on ways to determine patient competence.

18 **True or False** All the statutes in various states agree that any adult may execute a living will.

19 **True or False** Living wills are limited in the conditions under which they are effective and the treatments they may authorize to be withheld.

20 **True or False** Living wills must be executed in the same manner as a last will and testament.

21 **True or False** Health care workers should be concerned with criminal and civil liability for carrying out the wishes documented in a living will.

22 **True or False** The destruction of a patient's living will creates possible liability for a health care professional.

23 **True or False** Durable powers of attorney for health care decisions have broader applications than living wills.

24 **True or False** The advantage of a durable power of attorney is that an attorney always makes the decisions and family members are not involved.
25 **True or False** Durable powers of attorney for health care decisions appoint a particular decision maker instead of defining a particular decision.
26 **True or False** Durable powers of attorney apply only to decisions regarding life-sustaining treatment.
27 **True or False** When no advance directive exists and the wishes of the patient are not clear, life-sustaining treatment would likely be withdrawn.
28 **True or False** The same rules apply for patients in a persistent vegetative state as for incompetent patients.
29 **True or False** The same rules apply for persons who have never been competent as for competent patients who have become incompetent.

CRITICAL THINKING QUESTIONS & ACTIVITIES

1 What factors do you personally believe make life worth living? Defend your answers.
2 How many imaging professionals in your area have living wills? Talk to them and learn their reasons. Evaluate your own needs.
3 Make contact with chaplains and social services to review the types of services offered to patients with terminal illnesses.
4 Visit a hospice.
5 Do a case study on a patient who has received passive euthanasia.
6 Develop a list of criteria for establishing a plan for active euthanasia. The criteria and supporting factors should be recorded.

COST VERSUS SERVICE

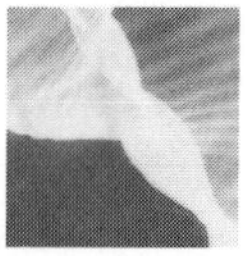

LIKE MOST IMAGING ADMINISTRATORS, I've often seen daily and even strategic operations boiled down to the classic economic argument of "guns versus butter." For those unfamiliar with this, the argument holds that choices are made between producers and consumers. These choices, in the most simplistic sense, are over whether to produce (consume) none, some, or a lot of a particular object versus another. Your choice or preference of one means that the other may suffer because resources are usually fixed and often limited. Such is clearly the case with health care today, and necessarily affects decision making of imaging administrators.

A classic example in our profession relates to the seemingly conflicting choices over level of service to provide versus the expense of that service. It is reasonable to be expected to use resources, labor, and supplies wisely. Even with the intense scrutiny and drive for increasing productivity, it is also reasonable to expect ongoing improvement in care delivery from a cost standpoint, specifically measured in cost per unit of service. As with cost measures and quality and service indicators, an administrator should strive to be in the best quartile of any given indicator in which reliable benchmarking information is available. Accomplishing all of this is at the very least quite difficult, particularly with the penchant of organizations to focus primarily on financial measures.

What can you do to at least strive to be one of those rare providers able to successfully balance cost and service? First, you'll lose the argument with financial officers every time if you don't come armed with good data, specifically quality and service outcomes as related to financial indicators. Don't shy away from comparative data—embrace it and seek the best practice strategies to improve both cost and quality measures for your operations.

Another important strategy relates to having solid respect for and application of process improvement methodologies. When one examines a particular process and focuses on improving its quality, costs decrease naturally. Real-life applications in which cost and quality are improved through process management abound in other industries; these techniques are slowly gaining a foothold in health care.

These two strategies, simple to grasp but more difficult to practice artfully, are basic to those rare administrators who provide good service at a reasonable price. The two do not have to be mutually exclusive; it isn't a choice of guns versus butter. A wringing of hands over the latest round of budget cuts does no one—patients, organization, or staff—any good. We can choose to be victims or we can choose to get assertive, prove our case, and work to better our cost position and our service levels. Low cost and high service? I believe we can have both.

JAMES D. MACE, MBA, RTCR
SENIOR DIRECTOR—PROFESSIONAL SERVICES
RIVERSIDE METHODIST HOSPITALS
Columbus, Ohio

CHAPTER 6

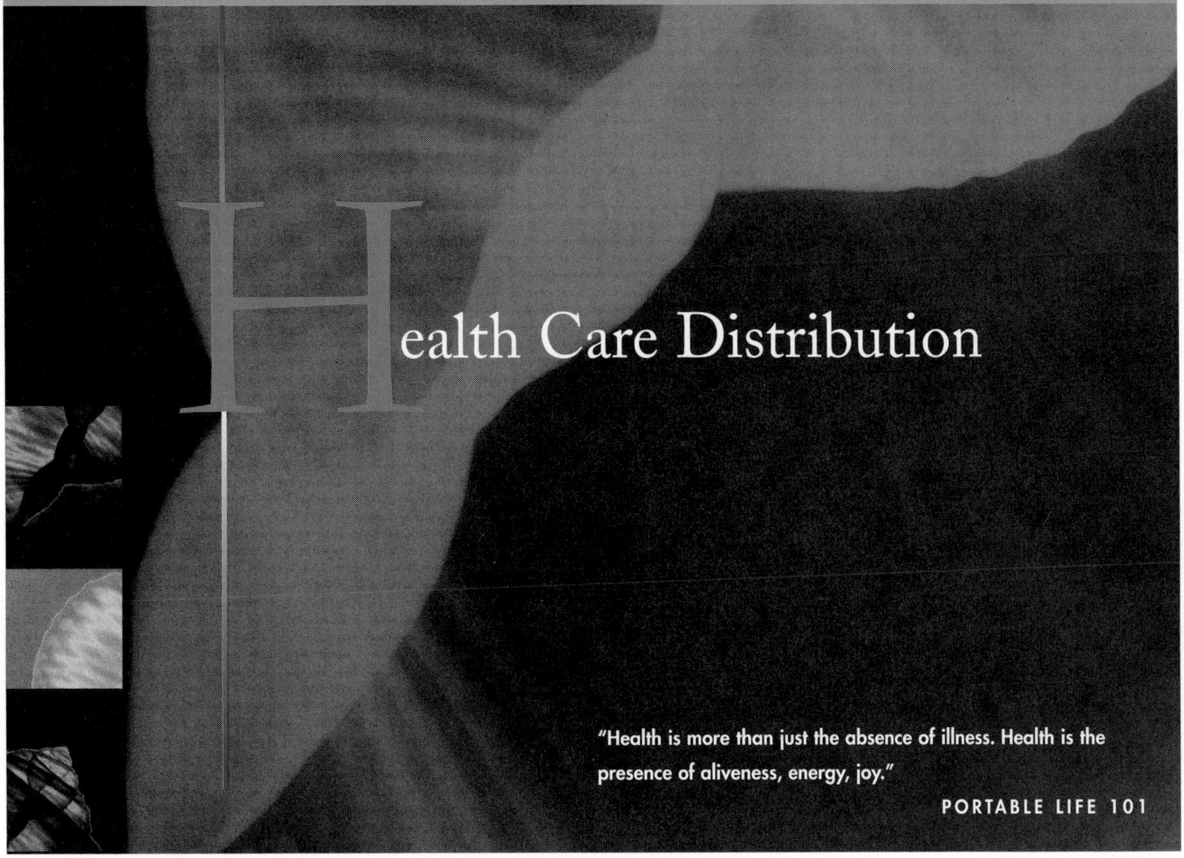

Health Care Distribution

"Health is more than just the absence of illness. Health is the presence of aliveness, energy, joy."

PORTABLE LIFE 101

LEARNING OBJECTIVES

- Evaluate the right to health care.
- Analyze ethical theories of distribution of health care.
- Describe managed care and its implications for imaging professionals and imaging services.
- Define *patient-focused care.*
- Integrate concepts of quality care and cost effectiveness.
- Recognize the imaging professional's role in health care distribution.
- Analyze the legal implications of cross-training in imaging services.
- Describe legal safeguards provided by proactive approaches to cross-training and streamlining imaging services.
- Recognize possible liability issues with regard to denial of authorization of testing.
- Define the possible roles of imaging professionals as patient advocates in managed care settings.
- Discuss the liability issues these roles may create.

CHAPTER OUTLINE

ETHICAL ISSUES

The ethics of health care distribution affects both imaging professionals and patients. Reform of the health care environment, services, patient rights, and the imaging professional's changing role in care all are topics that need to be addressed. The ethical challenges inherent in health care are changing, and imaging professionals also must be prepared to change. Changes require critical thinking, flexibility, and a continued desire to provide quality imaging services.

BIOMEDICAL ETHICAL CHALLENGE

Because of imaging equipment manufacturers' advertisements in the mass media, the public has become more aware of the quality of radiographic images and their diagnostic importance. As a result of this increased awareness, patients may begin to demand these new, expensive procedures. As such advertisements become more prevalent, questions regarding the ethics of health care industries marketing to target patients become more complex. Patients may feel entitled to the benefits of new technologies and may make demands on physicians and institutions to facilitate their needs. However, questions surrounding the reimbursement process remain controversial. The patient, provider, and third-party payer must come to terms with the availability of services and the amount of reimbursement available for those services.

During his presidency, President Bill Clinton stated the following[1]:

> We must set and keep our sights on three goals: controlling rising health care costs, covering every American with at least a basic health benefit package, and maintaining consumer choice in coverage and care. Putting people first in health care calls for a fundamental reform of the system. It requires that we combine an appropriate and revised governmental role with reliance on the private sector to provide care and to compete to serve every person in this country. But that competition must take place under a restructured set of ground rules that foster competition to provide the best care at the best price, not to avoid covering the less healthy and to raise prices fastest for the sickest.

These administrative objectives and the ways in which they affect the medical imaging services are having a profound impact on imaging professionals. The challenge is to provide more care with fewer resources in a demanding customer service–oriented environment while maintaining quality imaging services.

RIGHTS AND HEALTH CARE

Before a right to health care may be discussed, the terms *right* and *health care* must be defined. A *right* in this context means a just claim or an entitlement. Americans tend to believe that all people deserve health care as a matter of course. However, this may be a simplistic notion. Should all people, regardless of whether they pay for their health care, are homeless, or are financially irresponsible and cannot afford health care, be able to claim routine health care as a right?

The second term, *health care,* encompasses many elements. It may be perceived as a practice, a commodity, an approach, or a collective responsibility. *Health* may be described as a condition or frame of mind. All these definitions help inform a discussion of health care.

RIGHT
A right is a claim or an entitlement.

HEALTH CARE
Health care is a practice, a commodity, an approach, or a collective responsibility to ensure the wellness of a population.

To answer the ethical question of whether a right to health care exists, medical professionals need to ask whether health care is an element in autonomy and self-determination. Self-determination requires patients to participate in their own health care. Patients need knowledge, awareness, and continuing education regarding what they can do to maintain health to be full participators in their care. This is as important in the health care process as the provision of health care services. However, self-determination also requires patients to take responsibility for their health. Smokers who have chronic respiratory problems require many health care services, including chest studies, sinus radiographs, computed tomography (CT) scans, and other procedures. However, do such patients not bear some responsibility for their poor health? Should other patients suffer delayed access to imaging examinations because of the examinations required by patients who have not participated in their own health care? Should society pay the health care costs of those who do not take care of themselves?

SCARCITY AND DISTRIBUTION

Society is under many demands to provide health care for all citizens. The increasing costs of health care and the demands of a growing population place other stresses on an increasingly overburdened health care system. Nevertheless, many perceive a need for resources for the distribution of health care services to come from public as well as private sources, because "society is under an obligation to the individual to promote the common good."[2]

Resources in health care are increasingly expensive and scarce. "A sound theory [of] distribution, then, must provide for priorities and a system of allocating resources that at least regularizes expectations in the light of what is politically and economically possible."[2] Society, patients, and providers must make difficult decisions to aid in this distribution.

DISTRIBUTION THEORIES

TRIAGE
Triage is a system of prioritizing that encourages the routing of treatment to those with the greatest opportunity for a positive outcome.

Prioritizing, or triage, is an ongoing decision-making process in health care. The determination of which patient is the most important, is in the most critical condition, has the most need, or has the greatest opportunity for a positive outcome is an evaluation process necessary for the distribution of limited resources. However, triage is much easier to practice at an administrative level than at eye level with a dying patient. Triage seems to be a very practical method to bring justice and fairness to distribution, and society may see it as such, but it presents ethical conflicts.

The prioritization of patient needs influences the imaging modalities. Breast imaging scheduling often occurs under pressure by patients and physicians after a lump has been found. Many breast imaging suites examine patients every 15 minutes all day long, and many of these patients have to wait for diagnostic examinations after discovery of an abnormality. Prioritizing every patient's needs is difficult, and a number of theories have been advanced to aid the process (Table 6-1).

TABLE 6-1 THEORIES OF DISTRIBUTION: PROS AND CONS IN IMAGING SERVICES

Theory	Pros	Cons
Egalitarian	All persons have equal access to all imaging services	Patients' needs are different; scheduling and reimbursement would be different
Entitlement	All persons have needs	Patients must be involved in a contract to pay for services; theory more concerned with cost value of treatment instead of the intrinsic value of the service to the patient
Fairness	Balances dignity and equality of all persons with the inequality of their needs and circumstances	Identifying the differences (inequality of needs) can lead to subordinating the dignity of the individual to the convenience of the society
Utilitarian	Recommends providing the greatest good for the greatest number of people	Identifies patients as a group rather than as individuals

Egalitarian Theory

The egalitarian theory demands equal distribution of equal resources. This system believes every person is good and is equal. However, it does not address the fact that persons may not have equal needs. Moreover, whether this theory may be put into practice is uncertain. Carried to its logical conclusion, equal distribution of equal resources gives every imaging patient equal access to all imaging modalities. In what way would scheduling and reimbursement be handled under such a system?

EGALITARIAN THEORY
Egalitarian theory is a health care distribution theory that demands equal distribution of equal opportunities and resources.

Entitlement Theory

The entitlement theory sees the distribution of health care resources as a system of contracts. For this theory to work, a person must have a way to pay for the contract. The health care needs of the patient and the patient's ability to pay for required services do not fit into the value system to which some Americans are accustomed if those Americans believe they have a right to health care but are unwilling to pay for it. In addition, the theory seems more grounded in the financial value of medical treatment rather than its intrinsic value.

ENTITLEMENT THEORY
Entitlement theory is a system of contracts in which a patient has to pay for the contract.

Fairness Theory

The fairness theory tries to tailor health care distribution to balance the dignity and equality of all persons with the inequality of their needs and circumstances. The most important consideration in this theory is the ways in which advantaged and

FAIRNESS THEORY
Fairness theory is a health care distribution theory that adjusts the equality of individuals with the inequality of their needs and resources.

disadvantaged people receive care and who makes these decisions. Inequalities in health care distribution are frowned upon. "Identifying how these differences affect the person can easily lead to subordinating the dignity of the individual to the convenience of the society."[2]

Within this theory, the equality of patients as individuals is weighed against differences in their needs and circumstances. This weighing leads to a number of difficult questions. Do pediatric patients who come from financially disadvantaged homes have a right to an imaging examination their parents cannot afford? Should imaging procedures on individuals with mental disabilities be limited because of these patients' limited intellectual and financial resources? The fairness theory answers "yes" to the first question and "no" to the second. All patients are equal under the law and equal in human dignity, and regardless of whether they are unequal in means and resources, they still have rights to health services. However, difficulties arise in the determination of the degree to which a patient is disadvantaged.

UTILITARIAN THEORY
Utilitarian theory is a health care distribution theory that calls for realizing the greatest good for the greatest number.

Utilitarian Theory

As noted in previous chapters, utilitarianism recommends the provision of the greatest good (in this case, health care services) for the greatest number. Under this theory, imaging departments look at patients as a group and not as individuals and seek to provide the most care for the most people. Utilitarianism states that if a vascular laboratory can accommodate five uncomplicated procedures in one day, it should perform them instead of two long procedures. More patients are serviced in this way, and thus the greater good for the greater number is achieved. However, utilitarianism creates a number of problems. Individuals may have difficulty maintaining autonomy as the utilitarian theory is implemented.

RIGHTS THEORY
Rights theory is a health care distribution theory that claims individuals have a right to health care because of their human dignity and because society has an obligation to serve their needs.

Rights Theory of Justice

The rights theory of justice claims that individuals have a right to good health care because of their human dignity. In recognition of this dignity, society has an obligation to care for all people. This theory raises questions of rights and autonomy and the ways in which they are implemented.

PRACTICAL WISDOM
Practical wisdom is a product of right reason or virtue ethics that includes a consideration of emotional factors and development of the reason balanced by consideration of the consequences for the individual in society.

Practical Wisdom and Distribution

Another theory of distribution states the following[2]:

> Justice or distribution is accomplished through application of practical wisdom (right reason) to meet the demands of human dignity in the social circumstances of the time. Justice thus involves respecting human dignity and satisfying human needs and recognizing human contributions within the system and in ways that are characteristic of the system.

In other words, to serve the patient, imaging professionals must use practical wisdom to assess individual needs, ability to pay, scarce resources, and resource distribution. How are rights balanced with scarce resources? Who makes these decisions?

TRADITIONAL CARE

Traditional care allows patients the choice of their own physician and facility for health care services; however, the individual must be able to pay for those services. Each individual must have traditional insurance or be able to pay for the services. The more choices allowed to the consumer, the greater the cost of insurance. Traditional care provides quality health care for those who are insured with traditional coverage and for those who can pay for these services; however, those unable to pay and those uninsured find it difficult to obtain quality services.

Inequity of service, escalating health care costs, and demands from society have caused the United States health care system to become more sensitive to market forces. These factors have paved the way for the development of managed care.

HEALTH CARE DELIVERY MODEL/MANAGED CARE

Imaging professionals must define and explore the health care delivery model of managed care so that they may address the challenges reforms in health care distribution have presented to the imaging services. *Managed care* is an all-encompassing term that includes any type of system to coordinate the care and treatment of patients. Managed care is designed to provide better access, improved outcomes, more efficient use of resources, and controlled costs for the patient.[3] More simply, it is a general term referring to any type of delivery and reimbursement system that monitors or controls the type, quality, use, and costs of health care.[4] The aim of managed care is to reduce unnecessary or inappropriate care and reduce costs (Box 6-1).[5]

MANAGED CARE
Managed care is any type of delivery and reimbursement system that monitors or controls types, quality, use, and costs of health care.

BOX 6-1 WHAT IS MANAGED CARE AND HOW DID IT EVOLVE?

Management is the recognition, harnessing, and channeling of all available appropriate forces and resources toward meeting defined goals and objectives. What is "managed" in managed care? How a physician practices, among other things. Managed care is the application of management principles in a comprehensive, prepaid health care delivery system that controls input and output to optimize efficiency and effectiveness with the prior consent of providers and patients. In 1982, 10 million Americans were in managed care; in 1992, 90 million—a megatrend that continues to expand.

The alphabet soup of managed care includes IPA (independent practice association), HMO (health maintenance organization), PPO (preferred provider organization), POS (point-of-service plan), PGP (prepaid group practice), and the beat goes on.

The principles and practices of managed care are hardly new. The first group practice in the United States was established in 1887 at the Mayo Clinic and the first capitated plan was set up in Elk City, Oklahoma, in 1929. The Kaiser plan began in 1933 for employees and went public in 1947 as the first group-model HMO. By 1995, 56 million Americans were registered in HMOs, half of these in IPA-HMOs.

From Lundberg GD: Managing managed care, *JAMA.*

Whether managed care has accomplished these objectives is still to be determined. Not everyone has access to health care services, and whether the quality of care is increased or at least maintained at its previous level remains uncertain. Persons who were outside the system are still outside. Moreover, quality of care is perceived to be far down the list of objectives for most corporations; it is judged more by patients' perceptions of quality than by quality standards developed by the professional medical community.[5]

Managed care is having an impact on the ethical dilemmas faced by imaging professionals. It complicates the imaging professional's problem solving by adding questions concerning the needs of patients (both inside and outside the system), the medical community, and managed care corporations. Nevertheless, managed care is set to remain an integral part of the health care distribution system for some time to come[5]:

> Managed care takes many forms and is under so many different corporate structures that it is impossible to say it is categorically good or bad. The fact is that managed care is predominant in nearly every section of the country, and we must be able to adjust to the new way of providing patient care to our patients, making sure that we practice diagnostic imaging within the bounds of ethics.

PATIENT-FOCUSED CARE

Managed care is not the only model affecting health care and the imaging services. Patient-focused care also plays a significant role in the imaging professional's changing environment. Health care organizations and imaging services traditionally were designed to meet the fiscal needs of the organization. Now, following the lead of business and industry, they are currently developing and investing in services that address the demands and needs of the patient.[6]

PATIENT-FOCUSED CARE
Patient-focused care is a health care distribution model that calls for decentralization of patient care services and cross-training of health care professionals.

The primary objectives of patient-focused care are to move hospital care services closer to the patient's bedside and decentralize hospital services, including radiology services. Patient-focused care also seeks to implement teams of multi-skilled cross-trained health care professionals (including imaging professionals) to provide patient care.

The requirements of multi-skilling and cross-training for imaging professionals lead to ethical considerations that have an impact on imaging practice. Cross-training may require imaging professionals to perform functions that were previously performed by other health care professionals such as nurses and medical technologists. Critics of patient-focused care believe this cross-training and decentralization may lead to the loss of professional identity.[7] Critics also question the amount of training a professional requires to perform a variety of functions. This question leads to a consideration of the degree of competence an imaging professional must possess in other disciplines and the impact this competence or lack of it may have on the quality of patient care in the imaging services.

QUALITY AND COST EFFECTIVENESS

The new methods of health care distribution provide ethical challenges for all imaging professionals. Maintaining quality, providing access to more individuals, and cutting costs are problems for all imaging professionals. During this time of challenge and change they need to aspire to increase the quality of imaging services to maintain their professional status. The provision of more and better care with fewer resources requires sacrifice and planning on the part of imaging facilities. As medical imaging becomes more competitive and is forced to change, proactive facilities will thrive. They will be more cost effective, efficient, concerned with service, and driven by market factors. They will be survivors.[3]

Cost effectiveness may result from improved efficiency, empowerment of employees, and sensible delegation of duties. Efficiency may be improved by flattening schedules through elimination of peaks and filling in of low-use time. Cross-training employees to function in many capacities improves use of personnel. Wise application of automation also may improve efficiency.

Institutions may compete for cost effectiveness by determining their awareness of the efficiency of their services. This determination provides the basis for ensuring that patients receive the most cost effective and highest quality imaging services.

Imaging professionals and departments can help streamline performance by recognizing that they are in the service business. The focus of this business is the delivery of responsive, prompt, caring, and high-quality service.

Another way imaging professionals and departments can improve performance is by being aware of market considerations. The health care industry in general and medical imaging facilities in particular are under growing pressure to change. This pressure is driven by ever-increasing health care costs that must be borne by government, industry, and society. These cost considerations present a challenge to provide more cost-effective health care services without sacrificing the quality society has come to expect. Providing more cost-effective medical imaging in the face of evolving technologies that require more expensive facilities and equipment and more competent personnel is not easy. Imaging professionals will need to make the best use of their time, increase their productivity, and become multiskilled. They must be able to deal with change and be flexible in their assignments if they are going to enable their imaging departments to become more competitive, cost effective, and market driven. Facilities that become more cost effective will survive into the next century; those that cannot make this transition will not survive.[3]

IMAGING PROFESSIONALS' PARTICIPATION

Health care providers cannot be all things to all people or meet the needs of everyone. Choices regarding the distribution of health care must be made, implemented, and evaluated.

Individuals and society both have priorities for health care and must make their health care decisions based on them. These priorities are both intrinsic and extrinsic—the priorities people may personally hold may not be the same as the priorities they recognize for society. For their part, imaging professionals must remain continually aware of the problems and opportunities of health care service distribution. Hopefully, as imaging professionals develop a heightened awareness of the ethical challenges posed by changes in health care distribution, they too will be survivors.

LEGAL ISSUES

The American health care system is currently in turmoil. Reforms have been implemented because of two major problems: barriers that limit the access of many Americans to health care and the high and rapidly rising cost of health care. These reforms have brought about changes in health care that have had an impact on health care professionals, including imaging professionals. This section provides an overview of the ways in which the changes taking place in health care have a legal impact on imaging professionals.

MANAGED CARE

Managed care organizations came into existence to offer a more cost-effective way of providing health care. A managed care organization is a reimbursement framework combined with a health care delivery system, an approach to the delivery of health care services that contrasts with fee-for-service medicine. Managed care is usually distinguished from traditional insurance plans by its reliance on a single entity to coordinate both the financing and delivery of services, tasks that were previously performed by the insurer, patient, and provider.

Managed care is a growth area in health care delivery and is rapidly replacing traditional fee-for-service medicine. Managed care encompasses health maintenance organizations (HMOs), preferred provider organizations (PPOs), and independent practice associations (IPAs). Although the organization of these various groups differs, the concept is the same—the creation of a single entity to coordinate the financing and delivery of health care.

Much opposition to managed care has been voiced by physicians and patients. Physician opposition is twofold. The first problem involves the restriction of physicians' practice patterns by requiring pre-approval, sometimes denying diagnostic tests, monitoring drugs prescribed, and limiting the circumstances under which patients may be referred to specialists as well as the specialists to which patients may be referred. The second problem is the financial relationship of physicians with the managed care entities (Box 6-2). Patient opposition is generally based on the restrictions imposed on physician and hospital choices and a fear that they will become seriously ill and the plan will not come through with the best doctor or hospital (Box 6-3).

BOX 6-2 PHYSICIANS' OPPOSITION TO MANAGED CARE

Physicians have voiced much opposition to managed care. This opposition is twofold. The first problem involves the restriction of physicians' practice patterns by requiring pre-approval and sometimes denial of diagnostic tests, monitoring of drugs prescribed, and limiting the circumstances under which patients may be referred to specialists as well as limiting the specialists to which patients may be referred. The second problem is the financial relationship of physicians with the managed care entities.

Dr. Thomas O'Shea, a longtime Peabody, Massachusetts, pediatrician, witnessed the advent of HMOs in the decade before his retirement and grew to resent their interference. According to Dr. Shea, the HMOs limited when he could

From Bouchard K, Fitch MK: An ethical dilemma in the examining room, *The Washington Post,* November 17, 1996.

BOX 6-2 PHYSICIANS' OPPOSITION TO MANAGED CARE—cont'd

order expensive tests, monitored what drugs he prescribed, and told him what specialists his patients could see.

Shea says "You can only serve one master, and that's the patient. You can't serve a second master, and that's the insurance company. These HMOs come in and dictate what we can do. They got between me and my patients."

Another reason many physicians oppose managed care is the physician's financial relationship with these managed care entities. Under managed care, many doctors get paid up front by HMOs, which impose strict budget guidelines and scrutinize physician performance every step of the way. They also offer year end bonuses and other financial incentives that encourage doctors to keep costs down.

The growing influence of managed care has created an ethical dilemma for doctors, who, at least in theory, can make more money if they give patients less care. Whether or not doctors cave in to the pressure to limit care, the bottom line is that HMO cost concerns have invaded the examining room. Most physicians agree that good doctors would never deny necessary care, but they're still troubled by the questionable ethics of managed care.

Dr. Donald Hanscom, a Beverly, Massachusetts, gynecologist, says "It's very damaging to the doctor-patient relationship to have even the perception that doctors have a money incentive to provide less care." For example, Dr. Hanscom says, a doctor might encourage a patient to stay on birth-control pills rather than have a tubal ligation. At the end of the year, the money saved by not doing the operation would end up in the doctor's pocket.

Dr. Joseph Heyman, President of the Massachusetts Medical Society and an obstetrician/gynecologist practicing in West Newbury, Massachusetts, acknowledges the dilemma. Dr. Heyman says, "Primary-care physicians are sometimes put in the position of choosing between what's best for themselves and what's best for the patient. Fortunately, most doctors make the right choice."

To help physicians with this ethical dilemma, the Massachusetts Medical Society issued ethical standards for working within the managed care system. These include guidelines which make it clear a physician should never withhold care for financial gain and should disclose any financial incentives they get to hold costs down.

Modified from Bouchard K, Fitch MK: An ethical dilemma in the examining room, *Salem Evening News,* Salem, Mass. May 21, 1997, Essex Publishing.

BOX 6-3 PATIENTS' OPPOSITION TO MANAGED CARE

Patients' opposition to managed care is a good news-bad news kind of thing. Managed care members like the relatively low cost. But they dislike the restrictions on where care can be obtained.

A great example is Debra Thaler-DeMers, an oncology nurse with an insider's insight into managed care. DeMers held on to her fee for service insurance plan as long as she could. But when her employer, Good Samaritan Health Systems in San Jose, California, raised her monthly premiums to $220, $100 more than she would have to pay for Aetna Health Plans, an HMO, DeMers could no longer afford not to switch.

From Brink S, Rubin R: *U.S. News and World Report,* July 24, 1995.

Continued

BOX 6-3 PATIENTS' OPPOSITION TO MANAGED CARE—cont'd

Unfortunately, the oncologist who had been treating DeMers since 1983 for Hodgkin's disease (cancer of the lymphoid system) was not in the HMO. Their long-standing relationship and the fact that all the other oncologists that were in the plan were co-workers motivated DeMers to battle with the HMO over the issue. She even offered to pay the difference over what the plan pays its doctors. The HMO would not budge and DeMers began seeing a new oncologist, a doctor she works with every day.

DeMers, as an "insider," at least knew the quality of the care she would be receiving from her new oncologist. Many consumers, without that knowledge, fear that they will become seriously ill and the plan will not come through with the very best hospital or doctor. Some HMOs have contracted with regional specialty centers of unquestioned quality, such as for organ transplants or rehabilitation.

Despite the opposition, medical practice is increasingly moving toward managed care settings. They promise lower-cost care at a time when employers and the government are worried about the escalating costs of health care.

Managed care is here for the foreseeable future. To remain profitable, managed care must find ways to reduce the costs of providing medical care. This is accomplished by decreased use of testing, often through preauthorization requirements, and by contracting with facilities that can provide the lowest pricing. Health care facilities can provide services at lower prices only if they streamline their health care delivery systems.

REGULATION OF MANAGED CARE ORGANIZATIONS

Although the law regarding managed care organizations can vary somewhat with the type of organization, managed care is generally governed by both state and federal laws. Most states have HMO enabling acts, which address both the insurance and health care delivery aspects of HMOs.[8] A federal statute adopted in 1973 to encourage the growth of HMOs recognizes HMOs on the federal level.[9]

The federal statute imposes rules on HMOs that are meant to guarantee the provision of comprehensive health care. Under these rules, a federally qualified HMO must make health services available and accessible with reasonable promptness and when medically necessary 24 hours a day and 7 days a week and reimburse members for emergency services obtained elsewhere.[10] These rules also require services to be provided for a fixed premium, except for nominal cost-sharing amounts, deductibles for services rendered out of plan, and amounts collected from liability insurance or workers' compensation.[11] Safeguards are included to achieve fairness in premiums within groups.[12]

The federal statute also regulates the organization of HMOs, requiring them to achieve the following: be fiscally sound and make adequate provisions against insolvency; assume financial risk for the provision of services to their members (subject to reinsurance provisions); enroll persons demographically representative of the service area; accept Medicaid beneficiaries; not expel or refuse to re-enroll individuals because of health status or needs; provide grievance procedures; establish outcome-based quality assurance measures; make specified arrangements for members in case of insolvency; and develop, evaluate, and report performance statistics.[13]

State legislation authorizing and defining HMOs currently exists in every state but Hawaii.[8] These statutes vary dramatically, from a few brief sections in smaller states with minimal HMO penetration to pages and pages in states such as California and Florida, which have large HMO industries and have encountered serious problems with regulating HMOs.[8] HMOs are generally regulated by both the Department of Insurance, which oversees the insurer functions, and the Department of Health, which oversees the provider functions.[8]

A model Act was drafted and first proposed in 1972. It addressed many of the same concerns as the federal regulation.[14] Under the Act, HMOs must have a certificate of authority to do business in the state. The application for the certificate must be accompanied by a variety of information, including the following: copies of provider contracts; financial statements and feasibility plans; description of the grievance procedure and quality assurance plan; and a list of the providers with whom the HMO contracts.[14]

Additionally, under the Model Act, HMOs must perform the following[14]:

- Establish ongoing quality assurance programs
- Produce contracts that are not misleading or deceptive and contain a variety of information
- Provide grievance procedures for their enrollees and maintain records of complaints for review by the state
- Protect confidentiality of patient records and submit to evidentiary privilege and liability immunity for HMO peer review

Regardless of whether state HMO laws are expressly based on the model Act, they generally contain similar provisions. The most significant deviation is found with increasing frequency and mandates requiring HMOs to cover various types of treatment or treatment by various providers.[8]

PATIENT-FOCUSED CARE

As discussed earlier in this chapter, patient-focused care is another concept being implemented in an attempt to limit costs while providing better-quality care. Patient-focused, or patient-centered, care attempts to centralize patient services using the unit-based model seen with nursing care.

In the unit-based model, patients have a team of health care workers assigned to them. This can include a specific nurse, radiographer, laboratory technologist, respiratory therapist, social worker, and other allied health professionals. Under this model, the specific team assigned to the patient provides all patient care. Because the team provides all the patient care, members of the team may be asked to provide care other than that for which they were specifically trained.

WHAT DOES MANAGED CARE MEAN TO THE IMAGING PROFESSIONAL?

Both the managed care and patient-focused care trends have grave implications for imaging professionals. Under managed care, cost reductions are obtained through decreased use of testing, preauthorization requirements, and contracting with facilities that have streamlined their delivery systems to offer lower prices. If fewer tests are ordered, fewer imaging professionals are needed to perform those tests. If preauthorization cannot be obtained, and the HMO will not pay for the procedure, fewer examinations will be performed. Therefore if health care delivery systems are streamlined, imaging professionals may lose their jobs.

Patient-focused care uses allied health professionals, including imaging professionals, as a team to offer complete care to a particular group of patients. Under this system, imaging professionals may become involved in providing other patient services when their imaging services are not needed. They also may find themselves reporting to nursing personnel in their assigned unit.

To cope with the challenges of managed care and patient-focused care, survive professionally, and protect themselves legally, imaging professionals must strive to be proactive. Cross-training in another area is one way to be proactive, as is voluntary self-examination and improvement of efficiency.

Cross-training may have legal implications for imaging professionals, especially in the area of standard of care. When imaging professionals perform procedures in areas outside their training, they are held to the same standard of care as professionals trained and certified in that area.

Cross-training in another area and achieving certification are proactive ways in which imaging professionals may deal with the changes caused by managed care and protect themselves legally. If imaging professionals do not cross-train, they may find themselves in an ethical and legal dilemma if they are required or expected to perform procedures with which they do not feel comfortable. Imaging professionals in private practices may want to train as medical assistants or nurse assistants before they are forced to do so by the downsizing inevitable with managed care.

Imaging professionals also have the obligation and opportunity to scrutinize their own cost efficiency. If they can identify wasteful practices or wasted time, they can streamline their own practices before it is done by administrators who do not understand the imaging department. This allows control of the cuts to be made to stay in the hands of knowledgeable imaging professionals who can then make cuts where they will have the smallest impact on patient care. Voluntary self-assessment and improvement of cost efficiency allow imaging professionals to maintain more control over their own risk management.

Managed care may pose other risks for imaging professionals. For example, legal consequences may result when recommended treatment is denied by the HMO or PPO. Under managed care, more testing is performed on an outpatient basis. The interpreting physician reviews all ordered studies and recommends any additional procedures to be performed. However, the physician must first obtain authorization from the managed care organization or the facility will not be paid. Although liability for imaging professionals is unlikely, they may be drawn into litigation as witnesses if indicated treatment is denied.

IMAGING SCENARIO

You are a staff radiologic technologist in a small rural hospital. The department performs diagnostic radiology, computed tomography (CT), ultrasonography, and nuclear medicine. When nuclear medicine is busy, your supervisor often asks you to go and help. You do not mind this and have actually learned a great deal about nuclear medicine from observing the nuclear medicine technologist. Thus far your assistance has been limited to transporting patients, developing films, and generally assisting the technologist. The nuclear medicine technologist has never asked you to perform any patient studies.

One day the nuclear medicine technologist has called in sick with the flu, and the part-time technologist who generally fills in is also ill. Your supervisor approaches you and insists that you "fill in" in nuclear medicine. The emergency room has a patient from a motor vehicle accident on whom they have just ordered a liver/spleen scan to rule out a fractured spleen. Your supervisor explains that administration will be very upset if this patient has to be transported because radiology could not provide services.

You perform the test and the images look satisfactory to you. The radiologist interprets the study as normal, and the patient is sent back to the emergency room and eventually admitted for observation. During the night, the patient bleeds internally, is rushed to surgery, and a fractured spleen is discovered. Later, the hospital receives a request for the medical records from the patient's uncle, an attorney.

Discussion questions

- To what standard of care will your performance of the liver/spleen scan be held?
- Even if the scan were performed perfectly, will the fact that you were not certified in nuclear medicine have an impact on the legal outcome?
- Are state and national licensure issues evident here?
- Will this mishap affect facility accreditation?

Managed care case law is still in its early stages, but one court has found that the ordering physician has a duty to fight the managed care organization to ensure the necessary testing for patients. In *Wickline v State,* the court addressed the treating physician's obligation to appeal utilization review limitations.[15]

The case involved the postoperative release of a patient from a hospital in less time than the treating physician thought ideal. The plaintiff, Lois J. Wickline, alleged that the complete occlusion of the blood supply to the right leg that resulted in the amputation of that leg was caused by this early postoperative release. The treating physician had applied to Medi-Cal (the California Medicaid system) for an extension, had been refused, and had not appealed the denial. The patient sued the Medi-Cal program. The original court found that Medi-Cal was liable for refusing to follow the doctor's recommendation. However, the Court of Appeals reversed the ruling and found that the ultimate liability rested with the attending physician. *Wickline* suggests that the attending physician be aware of the third-party payer's reimbursement structure and engage in bureaucratic infighting when necessary, to the point of exhausting procedural rights, when the utilization review process has rejected a recommendation.

This physician liability is underscored by the fact that federal law practically bars lawsuits against HMOs. The Employment Retirement Income Security Act of 1974 (ERISA)[16] almost always preempts state law claims against health insurers for patient care and medical negligence lawsuits. States are attempting to create legislation to remedy this problem, but much opposition has been voiced from the insurance industry. Thus far, Texas is the only state that has enacted a statute allowing these claims. In the meantime, because physicians can be found liable, the door is open for them to be sued when health care is compromised because of denial of third-party payers.

What obligations do imaging professionals have if an interpreting physician recommends another study but the authorization for that study is denied? Must they communicate the seriousness of the recommendation to the ordering physician, so the ordering physician can decide whether to fight the denial? Although unlikely, the potential exists for patients to leave the imaging department with undiagnosed fractures, ruptured appendixes, fractured spleens, and other life-threatening conditions when authorization for recommended additional diagnostic testing is denied. Because of their unique relationship with patients, particularly outpatients, imaging professionals may be the only health care professionals who communicate with and observe patients sufficiently to recognize and inform the interpreting physician of the severity of the patient's symptoms.

IMAGING SCENARIO

A 28-year-old female outpatient with abdominal pain is examined in the radiology department. The treating physician's office has not seen the patient but has phoned in orders for an abdominal ultrasonographic examination. The examination is performed and is unremarkable. The ultrasound technologist, however, through communication with and observation of the patient, realizes that her pain is actually in the pelvis on the left side. The technologist also notes that the pain has increased in severity since the patient's arrival. These observations are passed on to the interpreting physician, who then recommends a pelvic ultrasonographic examination. The treating physician's office calls back to inform the technologist that authorization for the examination is denied, and the patient is to come into the office the next day.

Discussion questions

- Does this imaging professional have an obligation to act as an advocate for that patient?
- Could this imaging professional be subject to liability if the patient goes home and has an ectopic pregnancy that ruptures during the night?

Does the imaging professional then have an obligation to become a patient advocate? Is liability possible if an imaging professional sends a patient with serious symptoms home because a managed care organization has not authorized further testing? Although no case law exists on the subject, the standard of care of the imaging professional would likely create some kind of obligation to at least communicate concern to the interpreting or ordering physician.

SUMMARY

The right to health care is assumed by many in modern society. However, most also agree that with this right comes the responsibility for ensuring individual health care by implementing wellness programs.

A sound theory of distribution must be developed, accepted, and employed to facilitate patients' and society's growing awareness of health care issues. The theories of health care distribution include triage, the egalitarian theory, the entitlement theory, the fairness theory, the utilitarian theory, and the rights theory of justice.

Justice in health care distribution should involve "practical wisdom." Imaging professionals must keep in mind individual needs, scarce resources, and resource distribution when making health care distribution decisions.

Traditional care provides consumers with freedom of choice for health care services as long as they have the ability to pay for these services, either with health care insurance or on their own.

Managed care refers to any type of delivery and reimbursement system that monitors or controls the type, quality, use, and costs of health care. Its aim is to reduce costs, increase access to health care services, and improve patient care. Whether these aims and objectives have been accomplished remains to be seen. Ethical problem solving for imaging professionals has been further complicated by managed care.

Quality and cost effectiveness entail the provision of more high-quality health care with fewer resources. This objective may be facilitated by empowering employees, delegating, cross-training, and applying automation wisely. Institutions and individuals must provide high-quality customer service to ensure that patients receive cost-effective and high-quality imaging services.

Imaging professionals make daily decisions concerning the distribution of health care services. To survive in this changing environment, imaging professionals must develop a heightened awareness of ethical decision-making procedures in health care distribution dilemmas.

Managed care, in which a single entity coordinates the financing and delivery of health care, is here for the foreseeable future. Managed care has an impact on the imaging professional's practice through decreased testing, preauthorization requirements, and a demand for streamlined, lower-cost health care delivery.

Proactive responses to these changes will help imaging professionals continue to keep risks of litigation to a minimum. Cross-training and obtaining certification in other areas are proactive responses to changes in the health care environment.

Another response is voluntary scrutiny of cost efficiency and the implementation of appropriate changes, which allows the imaging professional to maintain control over decisions that have an impact on risk management.

Managed care can draw the imaging professional into litigation in other ways, especially in considerations of the duty of a treating physician to fight managed care organizations if necessary testing or treatment is denied. Although liability is unlikely for imaging professionals, they may be drawn into litigation as witnesses for or against ordering and interpreting physicians. The unique relationship between imaging professionals and patients, particularly outpatients, in such situations may place additional responsibilities on imaging professionals to become patient advocates.

ENDNOTES

1. Clinton WJ: The health care platform, *Adv Admin Radiol* 3:28, 1993.
2. Garrett TM, Baillie HW, Garrett RM: *Healthcare ethics, principles and problems,* ed 2, Englewood Cliffs, NJ, 1993, Prentice Hall.
3. Barnes JE: Batten down the hatches, *Adv Admin Radiol* 3:38, 1993.
4. Congressional Budget Office: *Effects of managed care: an update,* Washington, D.C., March 1994, U.S. Government Printing Office.
5. Folland S, Goodman AC, Stano M: *The economics of health and health care,* New York, 1993, Macmillan.
6. Strasen L: Redesigning hospitals around patients and technology, *Nurs Econ* 9(4):233, 1991.
7. Pack DA: Patient-focused care and the future of radiography, *Radiol Technol* 65(6): 375, 1994.
8. Furrow B et al: *Health law,* St. Paul, Minn., 1995, West.
9. 42 USCA Section 300e to 300e-17. See also C.F.R. Section 417.000-417.180.
10. 42 USCA Section 300 e (b)(4).
11. 42 USCA Section 300 e (b)(1).
12. 42 USCA 300 e(1), (2).
13. 42 USCA 300e; 42 C.F.R. Section 417.107.
14. NAIC, Health Maintenance Organization Act of 1990, Sections 3A, 3C, 7, 8, 11, and 28.
15. *Wickline v State,* 239 Cal. Rptr. 810 (1986), review granted and opinion superseded 727.P.2d 753 (Cal. 1986).
16. 29 USCA Section 1144(a).

REVIEW QUESTIONS

1 Describe four ways in which health care may be defined:
a. ______________________________
b. ______________________________
c. ______________________________
d. ______________________________

2 Resources in health care are increasingly ____________ and ___________.

3 List and describe the four distribution theories:
a. ______________________________
b. ______________________________
c. ______________________________
d. ______________________________

4 Critics of patient-focused care believe that cross-training and decentralization may lead to the loss of ______________ ______________.

5 List four ways in which cost effectiveness can be improved:
a. ______________________________
b. ______________________________
c. ______________________________
d. ______________________________

6 **True or False** An entitlement may be the same thing as a right.

7 **True or False** The egalitarian theory uses a system of contracts.

8 **True or False** Managed care controls the type, quality, and costs of health care.

9 **True or False** Cross-training does not require the imaging professional to function in areas other than imaging.

10 **True or False** Cost effectiveness and the maintenance of quality imaging services are the essence of customer services.

11 **True or False** Imaging professionals need not worry about liability when they are told to perform procedures for which they are not properly trained.

12 **True or False** The standard of care for an imaging professional in a particular area of imaging is that of a professional trained and certified in that particular area of expertise.

13 **True or False** Under managed care, the imaging professional can do nothing to control risk.

14 **True or False** The managed care organization is responsible for outcomes if they deny authorization for treatment or testing.

15 **True or False** Treating physicians may be found liable if they do not appeal the denial of treatment or testing they feel is essential.

16 **True or False** Imaging professionals may be involved in litigation as witnesses when additional testing in the radiology services is recommended and authorization is denied.

17 **True or False** Imaging professionals may have a responsibility to become patient advocates if they become aware of the severity of an outpatient's illness and testing is denied.

CRITICAL THINKING QUESTIONS & ACTIVITIES

1 Discuss the individual right to health care and compare it with the individual's responsibility for personal health.
2 Compare and contrast the theories of distribution and select the one you feel is most appropriate.
3 Develop a plan for providing more care with fewer resources in radiology services.
4 Explain the imaging professional's role in health care distribution.
5 Explain how justice involves respecting human dignity and satisfying human needs.
6 Identify your present state of wellness and initiate a plan to improve it.
7 Interview a health care provider who has come from another country with a different type of health care system such as Canada.
8 Evaluate the present cost effectiveness of your imaging area and develop an improvement plan.
9 Discuss any personal experiences with the health care/managed care system that indicate a need for improvement.
10 Select two teams to debate the managed care issue. Fact sheets should be created by each team to include areas of cost effectiveness, needs, distribution, and quality. Providing more care with fewer resources and maintaining quality should be the key factors of concern. Videotape or audiotape the presentation.
11 Discuss subspecialty areas available in your state for cross-training and certification.
12 Discuss the imaging scenario given in this chapter. Discuss options available to the imaging professional to deal with such dilemmas.

PROFESSIONAL PROFILE

EDUCATORS AND STUDENTS ALIKE must be well versed in the use of documentation to ensure due process. The importance of documentation within due process regarding student or employee issues cannot be overstated.

Student termination from an educational program for academic reasons is usually quite clear. In this instance a passing grade has not been achieved in a required course. Although termination may be an obvious consequence, due process requires that the student be informed at appropriate points (such as after midterms or other examinations) of the impending academic failure. Documentation that the student was informed is very important. Due process further demands that some documentation that the student was informed be made.

Student performance in clinical education is often the source of behavioral issues that must be addressed. In such a situation, both the educator and student should document points of contention. This makes conferences more meaningful for the student and more constructive for everyone involved. If the issue turns out to be a problem with clinical staff, student documentation of events is invaluable in communicating those issues to the clinical site. If the issue turns out to be student oriented, the student and the educator have concrete documentation from which to work. This could prove highly beneficial if remediation for the student is indicated. Documentation is the key word. It should focus on specific events, words, persons, places, dates, and times.

Documentation is the foundation on which due process is built. Conferences, oral warnings, and written warnings must all be supported by written documentation of the facts. This enables such warnings to effect the desired change in behavior. This change in behavior may be expected of the student, program faculty members, or clinical personnel. Without documentation and due process, personality whims and prejudices often replace clear thinking and resolution of problems.

Students often think that documentation is only used to affect them adversely. In fact, students can use documentation to their benefit as well. Occasionally, program directors and students must deal with disciplinary issues regarding program faculty members or clinical personnel. Students who are well informed on the need for clear, factual documentation and due process are often able to bring about the changes they need when dealing with faculty members or clinical personnel. Documentation may be used as the basis for conferences and to address serious situations that might otherwise be prolonged. Students have been able to ensure that their rights as learners and their dignity as human beings are protected by carefully documenting events and facts and presenting them to the appropriate authorities. Program directors have been able to rectify situations in which faculty members have caused emotional or mental distress to students that hindered the learning process. Students who are adept at documentation and due process graduate and become radiographers who make the workplace a more honest and unbiased environment.

CHAPTER 7

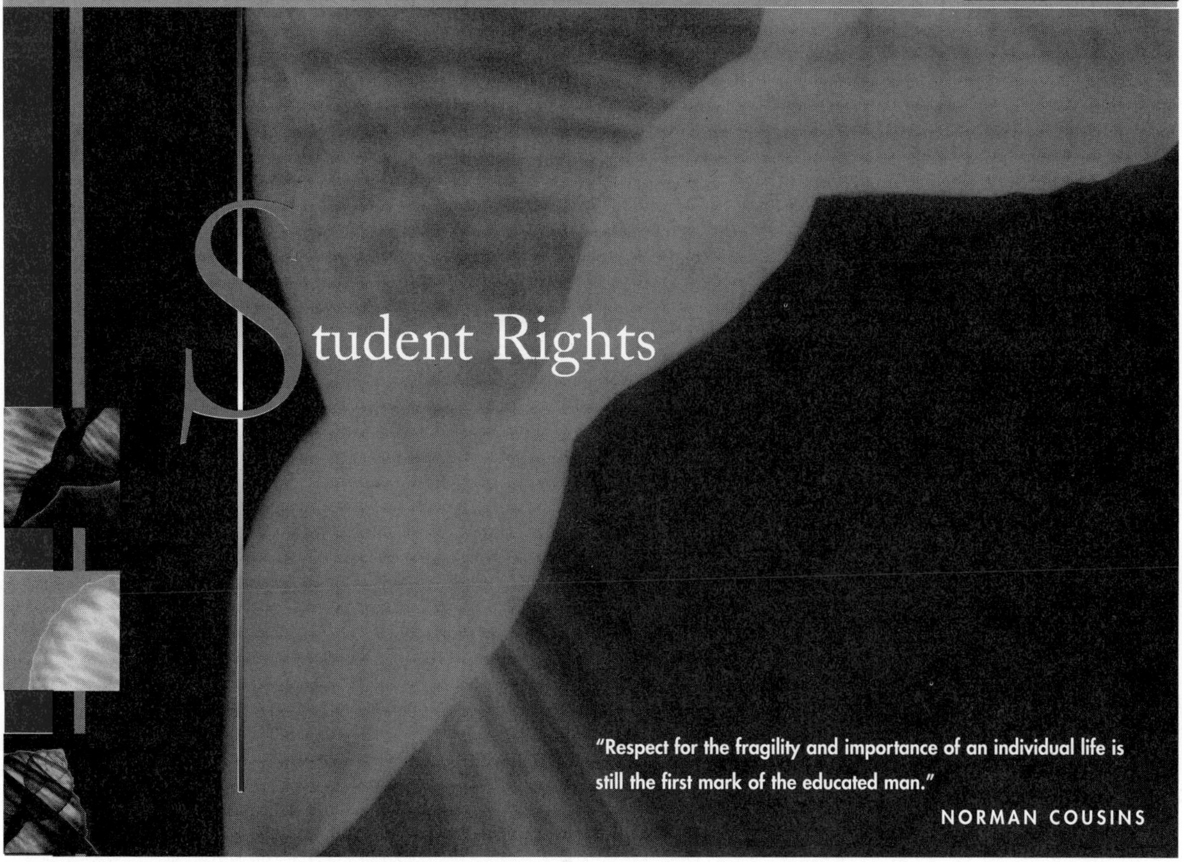

Student Rights

"Respect for the fragility and importance of an individual life is still the first mark of the educated man."

NORMAN COUSINS

LEARNING OBJECTIVES

- Explore the relationship between the imaging student's rights and ethics, including the following considerations:
  - Ethical theories and models
  - Autonomy
  - Informed consent
  - Truthfulness and confidentiality
  - Justice
  - Values
- Understand the legal doctrines affecting the relationship between the student and the education program.
- Explore the origin of due process.
- Define *substantive* and *procedural due process.*
- Explore the obligations of educational programs regarding restriction of student rights.
- Understand the procedural due process protections available when substantive rights are restricted.
- Explore the doctrine of employment at will.

CHAPTER OUTLINE

ETHICAL ISSUES

Ethical issues often come into play in discussions of the rights of imaging students. As prospective imaging students select and apply to the educational programs of their choice, and then progress through them, a variety of ethical dilemmas may present themselves.

Programs that teach imaging skills provide a variety of educational experiences. Each of the various modality programs offers unique opportunities for technologic, socialization, and human relations skills development. As the student develops each new skill, the opportunities for interaction and dilemmas regarding student rights grow.

Both imaging programs and students have concerns about student rights. They have ethical obligations to one another; these obligations later extend to the relationships among imaging professionals and others in the medical imaging environment. This chapter discusses these issues and provides examples of ethical dilemmas students may encounter concerning their rights during education.

ETHICAL THEORIES

The three ethical theories discussed in Chapter 1—consequentialism, deontology, and virtue ethics—serve as guidelines for ethical problem solving both for educational programs and imaging students. The choice of theory determines the basis on which each participant interacts within the educational environment (Table 7-1).

Consequentialism

Consequentialism evaluates an activity according to whether it can provide the greatest good for the greatest number. An application review committee at an imaging program may use this theory by selecting a large number of students with high

TABLE 7-1 ETHICAL THEORIES IN RELATIONSHIP TO STUDENT RIGHTS

Theory	Example
Consequentialism: the greatest good for the greatest number	Imaging students with the highest grade point averages may be selected to facilitate more educational opportunities for the group as compared to selection of students with lower grades who might require more teacher attention and progress more slowly through modalities
Deontology: formal rules of right and wrong	Formal rules may serve as a foundation of educational programs and policies regarding disciplinary processes and opportunities for students
Virtue ethics: holistic approach to problem solving using practical wisdom	Students may use intellect and practical reasoning when asserting their rights as students in a method useful to themselves and the educational program

grade point averages and significant clinical experience because this facilitates rapid comprehension of educational materials, thus allowing the students selected to include a greater variety of modality experiences in their education. However, student applicants with great desire to learn but lower grade point averages might consider this theory a roadblock to their goals of becoming imaging professionals.

Deontology

Deontology uses formal rules of right and wrong for reasoning and problem solving and judges an action on its merits alone, not on any possible consequences it may have. These formal rules may serve as the foundation of educational programs and student guidelines outlining student rights. A formal structure may be used to guarantee equal disciplinary processes and opportunities for students.

Virtue Ethics

Virtue ethics, a holistic approach to problem solving using practical wisdom, may play a significant role in the educational experience. Imaging students may determine that by integrating intellect and practical reasoning, they may assert their rights as students in a method useful to themselves and the educational program.

MODELS

Although ethical theories provide a foundation for problem solving concerning students' rights issues, the model of care employed by the program or student also helps define the ethical structure within which decisions are made (Figure 7-1). The model chosen—engineering, priestly, collegial, contractual, or covenantal—determines the ways in which interactions take place between students and educational programs. (See Chapter 1 for a more thorough discussion of these models.)

Students who feel as though they have lost their identity within the educational process may be working within the engineering model. An instructor who displays a godlike or fatherly attitude toward students may be employing the priestly, or paternal, model. A cooperative effort between students and teaching programs in pursuing the educational process is evidence of the collegial model. When students enter an educational program, they enter into a businesslike arrangement that defines the relationship between the student and the program. This is an example of the contractual model. After the contract, including aspects affecting student rights, has been agreed by both parties, an understanding based on traditional values and goals develops between the student and the program (see also *Contract Law* later in the chapter). This understanding is a crucial element of the covenantal model, which is based on trust and the experiences shared by the student and the program.

The model most often employed in imaging education is a combination of the contractual and covenantal models. A good example of this combined approach within the radiologic sciences is the learning contract in clinical education.[1]

As a result of the explosion in technology and the ever-increasing knowledge base required for clinical practice, programs are having difficulty providing students with all they need to know to function competently in a continually changing work environment. To facilitate the adequate education of students and prepare them for

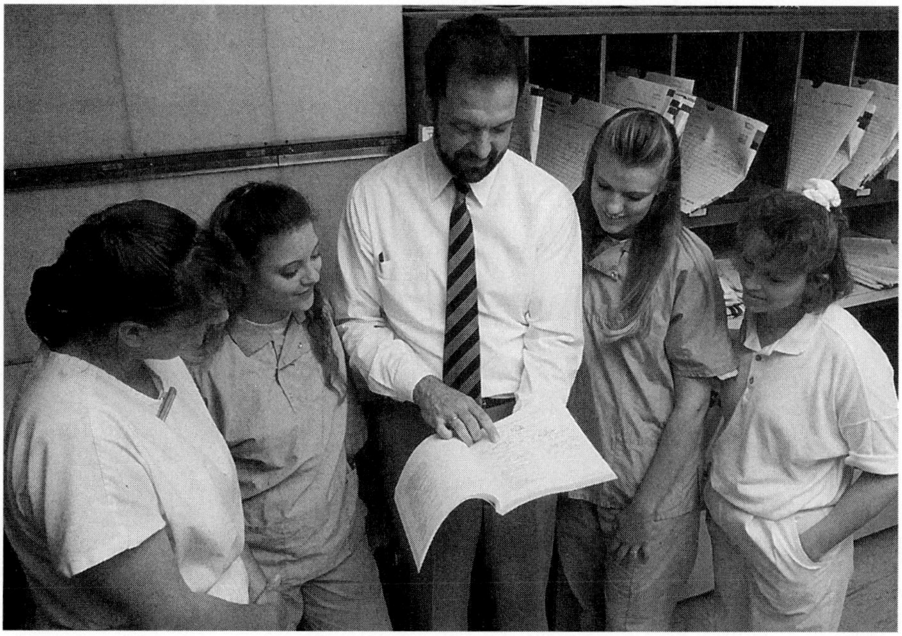

FIGURE 7-1
Students' rights involve problem solving.

employment in the evolving health care system, educational programs have developed learning contracts, which are formalized and mutual agreements between instructors and students that guide learning experiences.[2] Because they are contracts between programs and students, they require trust. Students enter the program trusting that they will be appropriately prepared to provide quality imaging services, and instructors trust that students are adequately motivated to uphold their responsibilities to study and perform their duties. When used properly, learning contracts may be valuable methods to provide needed experiences for students.[3]

Needed Imaging Experience = Students + Programs + Learning Contracts

STUDENT AUTONOMY AND INFORMED DECISIONS

The exercise and protection of student rights involve autonomy and informed decisions. The individuality of each student is an integral aspect of the educational experience. Each student has the right to be respected and treated with dignity and consideration. Students also have the right to expect quality education by quality instructors. Because student abilities and experiences differ, educational programs must be creative in classroom and clinical methodology.

Programs that respect student autonomy provide realistic and current employment opportunities for graduates. However, some programs that have noted poor results in their cost-benefit analyses face an ethical dilemma regarding employment. To maintain current faculty numbers, such programs may have to keep

BOX 7-1 QUESTIONS RAISED DURING COST-BENEFIT ANALYSIS IN THE IMAGING DEPARTMENT

1. Is student labor being exploited? Is the widespread use of student imaging professionals ethical?
2. Are clinical assignments being made fairly, ethically, and with an eye to keeping costs down?
3. Are education expenses for the program justified by the labor potential of the students?

IMAGING SCENARIO

In a hospital that has just experienced staff radiographer layoffs, a senior radiography student was assigned to the surgical rotation with a staff technologist. The staff technologist was sent home early because of a low procedure count, and shortly thereafter a disaster code was called. Several accident patients were arriving and some of them were going to surgery. The student was sent to surgery while the staff radiographers were busy with trauma patients in the department.

During the surgical procedure, the C-arm fluoroscopy equipment malfunctioned, and the student could not correct the problem. By the time the staff radiographer arrived to fix the C-arm equipment, the patient had died.

The surgeon was furious with the student and shared his anger with the other surgeons. The student was embarrassed and devastated.

Discussion questions

- What is the ethical dilemma?
- Whose problem is this?
- Are there remedies to this situation?
- How could the student have better dealt with this situation?

enrollment numbers at a maximum even if job opportunities are limited and graduates may face a very difficult job search.

The cost effectiveness of clinical education was discussed in a 1994 study.[4] It found that one of the primary concerns of administrators was whether the value of labor contributed by students offset the cost of educating them. Indeed, the use of student labor in clinical settings is an ethical concern for educational programs and imaging students contemplating their rights in the educational environment. If students believe they are being used in place of staff radiographers for cost savings to a department, they may question their clinical assignments. Moreover, educators may have difficult ethical decisions to make concerning student rotations if they feel pressured by administrators to facilitate greater student contact hours in the clinical setting. The rights of the students may be endangered if issues of cost savings by staff reduction are contemplated (Box 7-1).

BOX 7-2 REQUIREMENTS FOR INFORMED DECISIONS

- Information
- Attention
- Review

An emphasis on informed decisions encourages student autonomy by providing the prospective student with important information about the educational program and its policies and procedures. This exchange of information enables the student applicant to make informed decisions concerning participation in the program. After students have chosen and entered their programs, they typically are given a vast amount of information about their future didactic and clinical educational experiences. Educators should review this information periodically to ensure that students are provided with current and updated information that will help them obtain the skills and knowledge necessary to become qualified imaging professionals (Box 7-2).

TRUTHFULNESS AND CONFIDENTIALITY

Students have a right to the truth during the informed decision process, when they have a contractual agreement with the educational program. They also have a right to expect confidentiality during their education. Truthfulness and maintenance of student confidentiality are crucial elements in the relationship between students and instructors. Students put their trust in their instructors, who have the power to affect their future. They must be able to believe that when they ask even ethically difficult questions, they can expect the truth. A student who shares a personal confidence with an instructor should have the reasonable expectation that this confidence will be kept. However, this expectation of truthfulness and confidentiality may give rise to ethical dilemmas if the student expects to obtain truthful information that involves the confidentiality of another, or if the student makes a statement in confidence that may cause harm to another if it is kept secret. For example, a student may reveal a drug problem to an instructor with the intention of finding assistance and treatment. After a short period the instructor becomes aware that the student often works under the influence of drugs in the clinical area.

The instructor faces a dilemma regarding conflicting ethical obligations. If the instructor explains the problem to the program director, the confidence of the student will be betrayed. However, if the greater good is served, the violation of student confidentiality may be acceptable. In this case, from a legal perspective, quality of care and patient safety dictate a breach of the confidentiality between student and instructor. This situation should be covered in the policies and procedures of the educational program and the student handbook, and therefore the student should be aware of the consequences of such actions. These questions involve a balancing of student rights with the right of educational programs to maintain an appropriate environment for imaging education and services.

BOX 7-3 COMPONENTS OF A POSITIVE LEARNING ENVIRONMENT

- Truthfulness
- Maintenance of student confidentiality
- Justice
- Fairness

JUSTICE

A positive environment for imaging education also must encourage justice and fairness (Box 7-3). Justice in imaging educational programs is enhanced through appropriate application of ethical theories and models and the creation of an educational environment in which student autonomy, informed decisions, truthfulness, and confidentiality are valued.

Students expect to be treated fairly. However, fairness is difficult to define. One student's conception of fairness may not be the same as that of another. The following example illustrates the dilemmas resulting from differing conceptions of fairness.

A class of vascular imaging students is preparing for clinical evaluation. Each student has rotated in the vascular laboratory for 2 months and has had differing clinical experiences according to the procedures available. One of the students asks for an extension because the laboratory was slow during the student's 2-month rotation. The instructor denies the extension by explaining that the students were instructed to simulate procedures to practice when no actual clinical procedures were available in the laboratory. The student believes the situation is unfair because simulations are not the same as clinical experience. Is the student being treated fairly? What if all students demanded the same type and number of experiences before being considered competent? Such questions raise the issue of whether justice has the same meaning for all persons and whether a formula for fairness can be defined.

VALUES

A value is a worthwhile or desirable standard or quality.[5] Students and educational programs have particular values and standards that must become aligned for students to have a valuable educational experience. Student values motivate action and guide educational choices. Educational program values and standards are determined by organizational goals and mission. The values and standards of radiography and imaging programs also are determined by the Joint Review Committee on Education in Radiologic Technology Standards for an Accredited Educational Program in the Radiologic Sciences. These standards address a variety of issues important to students:

- Program mission and goals
- Program integrity
- Organization and administration

BOX 7-4 SOURCES OF ORGANIZATIONAL STANDARDS FOR IMAGING PROFESSIONALS AND DEPARTMENTS

- Personal and institutional values
- Joint Review Committee standards
- American Registry of Radiologic Technologists (ARRT)/American Society of Radiologic Technologists (ASRT) ethical standards

- Curriculum and academic practices
- Learning resources
- Student services
- Human resources
- Student rights
- Educational opportunities
- Students' physical safety
- Program fiscal responsibility
- Physical resources
- Program effectiveness and outcomes

All these issues are important aspects of the interactions between students and educational programs. They are discussed further in the legal portion of this chapter.

Another set of standards important to imaging students is the American Registry of Radiologic Technologists (ARRT) Standards of Ethics (see Appendix A). These standards are divided into two parts. The first part, the Standards of Ethics, serves as a guide by which registered technologists and applicants for the registry may evaluate their professional conduct as it relates to patients, health care consumers, employers, colleagues, and other members of the health care team. The second part, the Rules of Ethics, defines specific standards of minimally acceptable professional conduct for all presently registered technologists and applicants. They are enforceable rules intended to promote the protection, safety, and comfort of patients. Registered technologists engaging in any misconduct or the inappropriate activities listed in the Rules of Ethics are subject to sanction (Box 7-4).[6]

Students should understand and abide by the ARRT Standards of Ethics. They should be aware of the applicable standards when they apply for the registry, including those concerning moral turpitude and conviction of a crime. These standards remain in place despite the ethical concerns of educators and students regarding issues of confidentiality arising from these requirements of the certification body.

LEGAL ISSUES

Students entering educational programs for the imaging professions are taking a large and significant step into a new world that offers opportunities as well as legal and ethical dilemmas. An awareness of legal rights may aid students in their interactions with the educational program.

This section provides an overview of legal concepts that may have an impact on student rights. These concepts are defined in contract law and due process as provided for in the United States Constitution and state constitutions. This section also provides a basic overview of employment law, an important consideration as students become employees.

CONTRACT LAW

Students enter into a contract with educational programs. They should read such contracts carefully and be aware both of their own obligations and responsibilities and those of the educational program.

In general, contract law is based on the premise that parties can agree to almost any transaction as long as both parties know to what they are agreeing.[7] However, exceptions to this premise exist. One exception occurs when the bargaining power of the parties is greatly mismatched and the contract is grossly unfair to the party with less bargaining power.[7] In such a situation a court will not enforce a contract "which no man in his senses, not under delusion, would make on the one hand, and which no fair and honest man would accept on the other."[8]

This contract law applies to student contracts with educational programs and also to student handbooks, guidebooks, and departmental policies and procedures that establish the relationship between students and institutions. Unless a contract or the contents of a handbook or guidebook are grossly unfair to the student or program, the contract is valid and both parties must honor its provisions.

The validity of the contract between the student and the educational program, however, does not mean that disciplinary action can be taken arbitrarily or unreasonably. Every individual has certain guaranteed rights and among them is the right to due process in a disciplinary action against a student of a school or educational program. These constitutional guarantees exist in public and private institutions, schools, and colleges.[11]

DUE PROCESS
Due process as it pertains to schools outlines specific procedures that must be followed when disciplinary action is taken against a student.

DUE PROCESS

An important legal concept in education law is due process. Due process, as it pertains to schools, outlines specific procedures that must be followed when disciplinary action is taken against a student.[9] These guidelines must be followed to ensure fundamental fairness and reasonableness.

The Fifth and Fourteenth Amendments to the United States Constitution are the origin of due process rights in America. The amendment states that "no state shall deprive a person of his life, liberty, or property without due process of law."[10] This guaranteed right protects individuals from any legislative, executive, or administrative action that, in the court's opinion, is found to be arbitrary. If the court makes such a finding, the action is invalid. The policy and procedures manual for the program and student handbook should also ensure these due process rights.

In 1975 the United States Supreme Court extended due process rights to education, reasoning that the state, in creating the public school system, had created an entitlement it could not remove without due process.[9] *Goss v Lopez* involved the suspension of several high school students for as long as 19 days without a hearing.[11]

The court held that the damage to a student's educational opportunities and reputation caused by a 10-day or longer suspension was severe enough to require due process before imposition. The court further held that, except where a student's presence in the school presents a clear and present danger, notice and hearing should precede suspension and expulsion. Public and private institutions, schools, and colleges are subject to fundamentally fair procedural due process provisions with regard to a student's guaranteed rights.[11]

Due process, as defined by the courts, has two elements—substantive due process and procedural due process.[12] The substantive element defines and regulates the rights of citizens and defines the circumstances under which those rights may be restricted.[12]

The procedural element provides an opportunity for citizens to refute attempts by government to deprive them of their rights provided by the substantive element (substantive rights).[12]

SUBSTANTIVE DUE PROCESS

Dr. Michael Ward, while Chairman of the Joint Review Committee on Education in Radiologic Technology, related substantive due process to radiologic science educational programs. Substantive due process requires a school to show that denial of any of the student's rights to life, liberty, or property is a valid, objective, and reasonable means of accomplishing a legitimate objective. Additionally, any infringement on these rights must have a valid relationship to the improvement of the educational system.[13]

SUBSTANTIVE DUE PROCESS
Substantive due process is the notion that the rights of citizens and the circumstances under which those rights may be restricted must be clearly defined and regulated.

Ward uses an example to further understanding. Radiology programs commonly forbid students from wearing long, dangling earrings in their contact with patients. The fact that the director of education does not approve of long earrings is not a reasonable and valid condition for this infringement on student rights. However, if one of the school's objectives is to provide a safe and healthy environment for students in the clinical setting, and one of the means of accomplishing this is to deny students the right to wear dangling earrings because patients might accidentally pull them off, the chances of the school's meeting the requirements of substantive due process are much better.

PROCEDURAL DUE PROCESS

PROCEDURAL DUE PROCESS
Procedural due process is the mechanism by which citizens can refute attempts by government or other bodies to deprive them of their substantive rights.

After an investigation has established that a substantive right is being denied or infringed, procedural due process comes into play. Procedural due process, unlike some legal rules, is not a fixed concept but must be determined by the circumstances at hand.[14] The United States Supreme Court invoked a balancing formula to determine the exact procedural safeguards needed in a particular context.[14] According to

Ward, in the context of denying students' rights in a radiologic sciences educational program, authorities must provide at least the following[14]:

1. A written statement regarding the reasons for the proposed action
2. Formal notice of a hearing where the student may answer the charges
3. A hearing at which both sides may present their case and any rebuttal evidence

The procedure is not fixed, as stated previously. However, the process must be commensurate with the length of the suspension or the detriment that may be imposed on the student.

According to Ward, the administration of discipline should guarantee procedural fairness to an accused student. The educational institution has an obligation to clarify standards of behavior it considers essential to its educational mission and community life. Schools should avoid imposing limitations on students that have no direct relevance to their education.[13]

Ward further states that disciplinary proceedings should be instituted only for violations of standards of conduct formulated with significant student and faculty participation and published in advance through student handbooks or a generally available body of institutional regulations. If the misconduct results in serious penalties and accused students question the fairness of the disciplinary action, they should be granted on request the privilege of a hearing before a committee. The only legal concern regarding the composition of the hearing committee is that no conflict of interest or bias exists. Impartiality is the essence of fair judicial treatment.[13]

Ward points out the specific elements of procedural due process regarding hearings involving students. They include the following[13]:

1. Accused students must receive notice of the time and place of the hearing, as well as the charges and specific grounds against them.
2. Students must have an opportunity to be heard and must know the evidence against them.
3. The allegations against a student must be presumed untrue until they are found to be true by direct, competent evidence of misconduct. This presumption that the allegations are untrue allows accused students to remain silent during disciplinary proceedings without such silence being held against them.
4. Students' status should not be altered pending action on any charges, nor their right to attend classes or be present on the campus or in the clinic, except for reasons related to their own or others' physical or emotional safety.

Furthermore, according to Ward, other fundamental rights of the accused include the issuance of written findings of fact and the right to an appeal. These findings of fact should ensure that the hearing committee makes a decision based only on clear and convincing evidence presented at the hearing.

Legally, schools do not have to provide an appeal process. However, the *Essentials and Guidelines of an Accredited Program for the Radiographer* of the Joint Review

Committee on Education in Radiologic Technology provides that an appeal process should be defined and available to students.[15] Legally, judicial review is available to students to determine whether the hearing body violated their rights.

Appeals procedures help ensure that the student's interests are balanced against the school's sometimes contrary interests. Fairness and reasonableness should be the basis of the outcome of any such procedures.

The guidelines set out previously should be included in the policies and procedures of the program, handbook, and contract. These set out the guidelines to be followed by both parties. They also create an opportunity for the parties to sign off on these procedures, signaling their acceptance.

EMPLOYEE RIGHTS

A different set of rules governs the employment relationship. Health care workers, including imaging professionals, working in private health care facilities without employment contracts are generally subject to a legal doctrine called *employment at will.*

Employment at will allows employers and employees to terminate their relationship for no cause, subject to the restrictions of antidiscrimination and other statutes. This doctrine varies considerably among the states, but some generalizations may be made.[16]

EMPLOYMENT AT WILL

Employment at will is a policy that allows employers and employees to terminate their relationship for no cause, subject to the restrictions of antidiscrimination and other statutes. The concept of an implied contract provides an exception to the policy, as does the public policy exception.

EXCEPTIONS

Employees at will may have a claim for wrongful discharge if their situation falls within one of the exceptions to at-will employment in the jurisdiction. However, none of these exceptions has developed a position that health care workers should have special exceptions from the at-will doctrine.[16]

Implied contract is the most common exception to the at-will doctrine. This doctrine allows an employee handbook or personnel manual to be perceived as an enforceable contract. In such situations the court reviews the handbook or manual to determine whether it represents a contract and whether that contract prohibits discharge of the employee.[16]

The second most common exception to the at-will doctrine is the public policy exception, which allows for a claim of wrongful discharge if the plaintiff is discharged for conduct protected by specific state mandates.[16] This exception is quite narrow, generally requiring identification of a specific statute or state law that has been violated. Examples of the public policy exception include when discharge is in retaliation for the filing of a workers' compensation claim or because an employee served on jury duty against the employer's wishes. Courts have generally been unwilling to recognize a public policy exception for health care workers who claim they were discharged for criticizing or taking steps to improve the quality of patient care or for actions the employee claims were based on personal moral principles.[16]

As stated briefly previously, employment at will is subject to restrictions imposed by antidiscrimination statutes. These statutes are discussed in Chapter 8.

IMAGING SCENARIO

An imaging professional who has recently moved to town is hired to perform general diagnostic procedures. As is generally the case, no contract of employment exists. The imaging professional is very critical of the way things are done at the facility that has hired her. She repeatedly refers to the facility in which she previously worked, insisting things should be done as they were there. On several occasions, she ignores the policies and procedures of her current employer and performs procedures according to the policies and procedures of her previous employer.

She is counseled and written up for these infractions according to the personnel policies in the employee handbook. When her conduct does not change, she is terminated. She thinks this grossly unfair and seeks legal advice, stating that she was merely trying to improve the quality of patient care and do things the way they should be done.

Discussion

Employment at will

This employee is likely an employee at will because no employment contract was entered into.

Exceptions to employment at will

She argues that the employee handbook should be construed as an implied contract and she therefore falls under an exception to employment at will. However, even if the employee handbook can be construed as an implied contract, it contains provisions for the discharge of employees under certain situations. As long as the facility followed those procedures, including counseling and written reprimands, discharge is allowed.

She also argues that she was merely trying to improve the quality of patient care and her way was the better way to do things. Such an exception would have to fall under the public policy exception to employment at will. Courts have recognized these exceptions in very limited circumstances; these circumstances do not include a health care worker trying to improve patient care.

SUMMARY

Student rights are partially determined by the imaging student's and program's choices of ethical theories and models. Each theory and model provides problem-solving techniques and helps guide interactions between students and educational programs.

Autonomy and informed decisions are important elements in considerations of student rights. An informed decision process allows students access to information concerning application requirements for the program and other information necessary for appropriate imaging education. This process helps maintain student autonomy. Knowledge is important to the maintenance of the "self" of the student.

Mutual truthfulness and confidentiality enable students and educational programs to trust one another. Students have a right to expect confidentiality regarding their personal communications and records as long as this does not cause harm to another.

Justice or fairness is sometimes difficult to determine in an imaging program. Actions that seem fair to one student may seem unfair to another. In such situations, ethical problem solving using appropriate theories and models becomes important to imaging students.

Values and standards are desirable qualities imaging students should use in making goals for themselves in their personal and professional lives. The Joint Review Committee on Education in Radiologic Technology and the guidelines put forth by the ARRT provide standards and ethical guidelines for educational programs, students, and imaging professionals.

The legal rights of students in radiologic science educational programs are generally based on contract law and due process. Unless the contract is grossly unfair to the student, it is valid and both the student and the educational program have obligations to fulfill its provisions.

Due process is a right of all American citizens that originated in the Fifth and Fourteenth Amendments to the United States Constitution. In 1975 the United States Supreme Court held that this right extends to students. Due process has two elements—substantive due process and procedural due process.

Substantive due process requires radiologic science education programs to avoid placing restrictions on students that have no direct relevance to their education. After an investigation has established that restrictions on a student's substantive rights have been made, procedural due process requires procedural safeguards. These include the following: a written statement regarding the reasons for the proposed action, formal notice of a hearing in which the student may answer the charges, and a hearing at which both sides may present their case and rebuttal evidence.

The educational institution has an obligation to clarify the standards of behavior it considers essential to the educational program. Disciplinary proceedings should be initiated only for violations of standards that have been formulated and published in advance in student handbooks or generally available institutional regulations. If the misconduct may result in serious penalties and accused students question the fairness of the action, they should be entitled to a hearing before an unbiased committee.

The procedural process of such a hearing must include the following:

- The accused student receives notice of the time and place of the hearing and the specific charges.
- Accused students must have an opportunity to be heard and know the evidence against them.
- Students must be presumed innocent and their silence must not be used against them.
- Student status should not be altered unless a threat to the student's or others' safety is evident.

Written findings must be issued, and the student should be granted the right to an appeal. Judicial review is always available to students to determine whether the hearing body violated their rights.

The rules regarding fair employment are different from the rules of education. Employment at will is the legal doctrine that covers imaging professionals in private health care facilities without employment contracts. *Employment at will* means employers and employees may terminate the employment relationship at any time for any reason. Exceptions to this doctrine include antidiscrimination statutes, the implied contract exception, and the public policy exception.

Antidiscrimination statutes are discussed in Chapter 8. The implied contract exception allows an employee handbook or personnel manual to be considered a contract for employment. In any dispute, the court reviews the document in question to determine whether it represents a contract and whether that contract prohibits discharge. The public policy exception allows for claims of wrongful discharge for conduct allowed by specific state statutes or mandates.

ENDNOTES

1. Renner JJ, Stritter F, Wong H: Learning contracts in clinical education, *Radiol Technol* 64(6):358, 1993.
2. Knowles M: *Self-directed learning: a guide for learners and teachers,* Chicago, 1975, Follett.
3. Knowles M: *Using learning contracts,* San Francisco, 1986, Jossey-Bass.
4. Ballinger PW, Diesen MS: The cost effectiveness of clinical education, *Radiol Technol* 66(1):41, 1994.
5. Rokeach M: *Beliefs, attitudes, and values,* San Francisco, 1968, Jossey-Bass.
6. The American Registry of Radiologic Technologists: Annual report to registered technologists, St. Paul, Minn., April 1997, Author.
7. Dawson J, Harvey W, Henderson S: *Cases and comments on contracts,* Minola, NY, 1990, Foundation.
8. *Hume v United States,* 132 U.S. 406 (1889).
9. *Goss v Lopez,* 419 U.S. 565 (1975).
10. The Constitution of the United States of America, Amendment 14, Section 1, 1868.
11. Mawdsley RD: *Legal problems of religious and private schools,* ed 3, Topeka, Kansas, 1995, National Organization on Legal Problems of Education.
12. Rotunda R, Novak J: *Treatise on constitutional law,* ed 2, St. Paul, Minn., 1992, West.
13. Ward M: Due process of law and student rights, *Radiol Technol* 65(3):187, 1994.
14. *Mathews v Eldridge,* 424 U.S. 319 (1976).
15. Joint Review Committee on Education in Radiologic Technology: *Essentials and guidelines of an accredited program for the radiographer,* Chicago, 1990, Author.
16. Furrow B et al: *Health law,* St. Paul, Minn., 1990, West.

REVIEW QUESTIONS

1 Both ________________ and ____________________ have concerns about student rights.
2 ____________ provide guidelines for interactions between students and educational programs.
3 The ethical model used to facilitate the learning contract is a combination of the __________ and ________ models.
4 Autonomy includes which of the following?
 a. The self
 b. Informed consent
 c. Respect
 d. All of the above
5 The provision of a trusting environment for imaging students requires ____________________ and ______________________ .
6 Another term for fairness is ___________ .
7 Define *standards.*
8 List two organizations that provide standards for imaging students.
9 Give an example of the use of each model of care within the clinical setting.
10 What is the origin of due process law?
11 List and define the two elements of due process law.
12 When a school takes disciplinary action against a student, what actions do procedural due process require?
 a. ______________
 b. ______________
 c. ______________
13 Define and describe the legal employment doctrine that applies to most health care workers.
14 List the exceptions to employment at will.
15 **True or False** The cost effectiveness of imaging programs may provide educators and students with ethical dilemmas.
16 **True or False** Contract law prohibits parties from making unfair contracts.
17 **True or False** Contracts between students and educational programs may include student handbooks and guidebooks.
18 **True or False** A contract is valid even if it is grossly unfair to one of the parties.
19 **True or False** If a student's contract is valid, educational institutions can take any disciplinary actions they desire.
20 **True or False** Substantive due process defines the rights of citizens and the circumstances under which they may be restricted.
21 **True or False** Procedural due process applies regardless of whether substantive rights are affected.
22 **True or False** Educational programs may restrict student rights in any way they like.
23 **True or False** Educational programs have an obligation to clarify behavioral standards essential to the educational program.

24 True or False Standards of conduct cannot be published in student handbooks or institutional regulations.

25 True or False Hearings may be held by committees composed entirely of educators and the program director.

26 True or False If students do not speak at hearings to defend themselves, their silence may be used against them.

27 True or False A student is entitled to a written finding of facts from a hearing.

28 True or False Factors other than those presented at the hearing may be used in the decision-making process of the hearing.

29 True or False If the hearing committee finds the student guilty of misconduct, the student has no other options but to accept the penalty.

30 True or False The same rules govern employment and educational programs.

31 True or False Employers cannot discharge employees except if they find misconduct.

CRITICAL THINKING QUESTIONS & ACTIVITIES

1 How does motivation guide student choices?

2 Which ethical theory do you believe protects student rights to the greatest degree? Why do you believe this?

3 Provide a scenario regarding the lack of student autonomy caused by a poor informed decision-making process. Discuss your reasoning.

4 Describe a situation in which the truth may be a detriment to student rights. Defend your answer.

5 Define *fairness*. Is fairness the same for all students? Provide examples to support your answer.

6 What role did your values play as you explored your educational opportunities? Did your personal values ever come into conflict with the educational program's standards? Why do you think this occurred? What alternatives could have been implemented to rectify the situation?

7 How do you feel about the issue of sanctions being imposed on technologists who make statements in confidence to educators? How would you feel if you were the person involved in the process? How would you react if you believed your confidentiality was being infringed?

I AM THE PATIENT

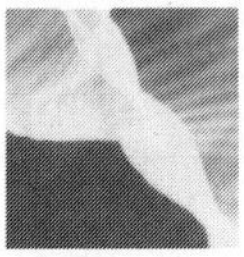

YOU'VE SEEN ME a hundred times . . . with many faces . . . many forms . . . many reasons for being in your care.

I am the frightened, middle aged woman waiting at your reception desk, nervously opening and closing her purse.

I am the shuffling, stoop-shouldered figure in the faded flannel you encounter as you go about your daily work.

Everything is new and strange to me. From the moment I walk up to your reception desk, I am a mass of fears. I am fearful of the unknown. I am alarmed over the prospect of pain, or radiation exposure . . . even death. More than anything else, I am lonely.

When I complain about the cold, hard table, I am trying to tell you of far deeper needs. Will I lose my identity? Will I be exposed to all sorts of indignities?

I'm afraid that I will not be treated as a housewife . . . but as a fascinating gallbladder . . . an interesting thyroid.

Though I am mature, I have suddenly become a child, frightened of the enormous machine whirring above my head. And . . . oh, how I want to be warm and friendly!

I want you to know that I bring with me a personality, not just another problem in your work . . . a vein that's hard to find . . . a chest that needs repeating.

I am suddenly hypersensitive. In spite of all your physical comforts, your padded waiting chairs, the soft music, I can be devastated by a blunt word from the technologists.

It may be that my sensitivity is exaggerated, but make me feel welcome. Tell me by your attitude that you respect me as an individual.

Much of my fright comes from lack of understanding on my part. All too often you take it for granted that I know things and I'm left to grope for my answers alone.

Help me bridge my feelings of embarrassment at the lack of privacy. Assure me that my dignity as a person will be respected.

Never forget, you're the symbol to people like me ever since the Samaritan traveled the road between Jerusalem and Jericho two thousand years ago.

The equipment and the methods have changed, but the concept continues unchanged. You're the benevolent healer. You cannot . . . Dare not . . . Change!

ELEANOR McMARTIN

CHAPTER 8

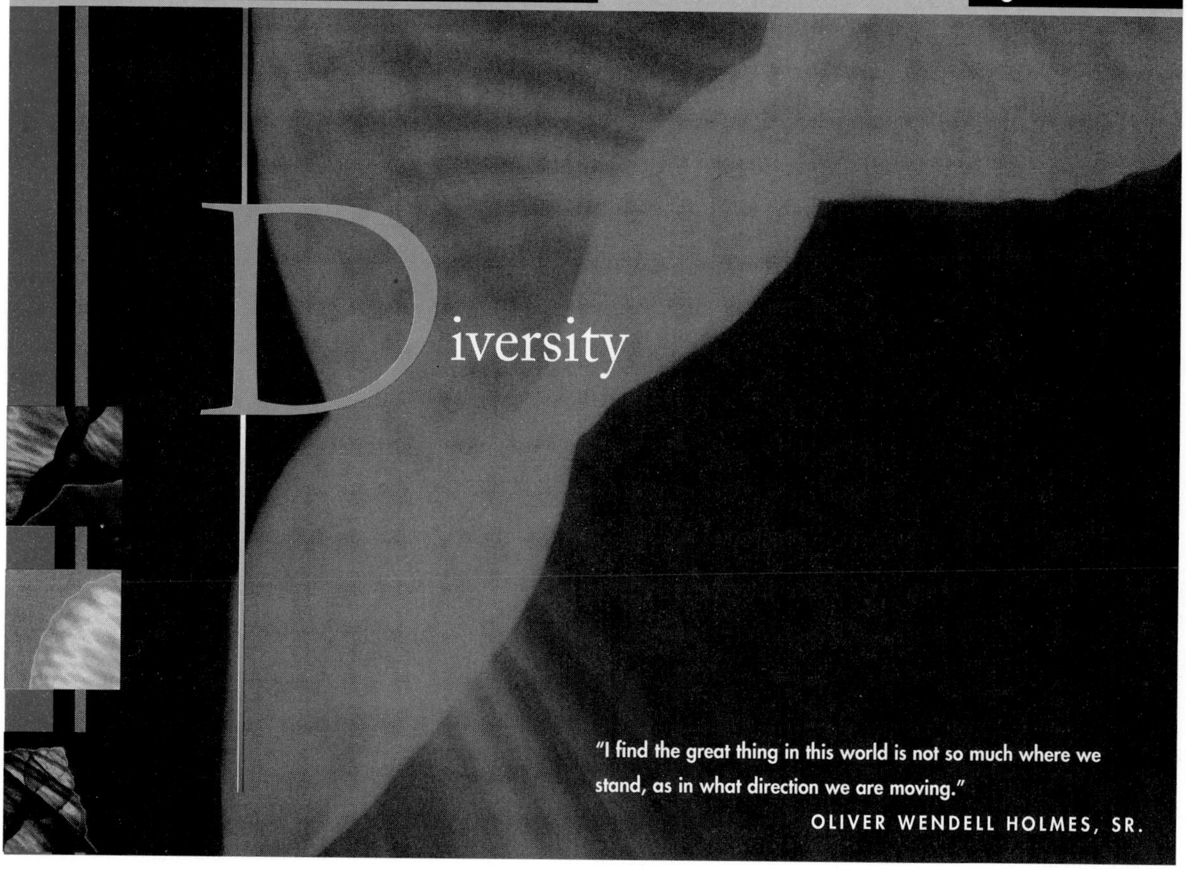

Diversity

> "I find the great thing in this world is not so much where we stand, as in what direction we are moving."
>
> OLIVER WENDELL HOLMES, SR.

LEARNING OBJECTIVES

- Define *diversity* and describe interaction patterns.
- Evaluate a study in diversity.
- Explain the ways in which diversity and ethical problem solving relate to each other.
- Discuss the ways values affect issues of diversity.
- Understand and discuss the origins of discrimination law.
- Explore discrimination law in employment and patient treatment solutions.
- Identify the two types of sexual harassment.
- Define sexually harassing behavior.
- Discuss the prima facie case of employment discrimination and hostile work environment, including sexual harassment.
- Understand and discuss the law regarding discriminatory patient treatment.

CHAPTER OUTLINE

ETHICAL ISSUES

Imaging students must prepare themselves for a variety of experiences, interactions, and problem solving in their careers. Every patient and situation is unique. This uniqueness may lead to dilemmas requiring imaging professionals to employ ethical problem-solving skills.

Imaging professionals, as well as other health care professionals, should be able to identify and accept differences among people. These differences include much more than skin color or native language. Imaging professionals must be knowledgeable about patient attitudes and perceptions regarding imaging procedures. Their mission is not to change patients so that they are all similar but to better understand the differences of their patients as they go about their work.[1]

Imaging professionals should develop their interpersonal qualities at all educational levels. Educational programs should emphasize an appreciation and respect for diversity. According to the proceedings from the American Society of Radiologic Technologists (ASRT) National Education Consensus,[2] issues of diversity will have an increasing impact on the imaging profession into the next century.

Imaging professionals are challenged to provide imaging services to individuals and groups of people with diverse expectations, values, and backgrounds. They must be flexible in their approach—no single method of providing imaging services to a diverse patient population with differing ideas about what constitutes "caring" is the best. Imaging professionals must be creative and innovative in providing acceptable, high-quality care for diverse patient populations. This chapter is devoted to defining diversity and enhancing understanding of its relationship to ethical problem solving.

DIVERSITY DEFINED

Within this chapter, *diversity* is not defined merely as a variety of ethnicities. Rather, it includes differences that may be rooted in culture, age, experience, health status, gender, sexual orientation, racial identity, mental abilities, and other aspects of sociocultural organization and socioeconomic position.[3] Issues in diversity may be divided into primary and secondary dimensions.[4] Primary dimensions include physical and mental health, sexual orientation, age, ethnicity, and gender. Secondary dimensions include income, marital status, geographic location, education, and religion.

DIVERSITY
Diversity is differences rooted in culture, age, experience, health status, gender, sexual orientation, racial or ethnic identity, mental abilities, and other aspects of sociocultural description and socioeconomic status.

The encouragement of diversity is an inclusive process of appreciation of the unique contributions different individuals with differing backgrounds bring to an organization.[4] For example, an educational program encouraging diversity values the differences among students and asserts that their uniqueness contributes to the formation of more knowledgeable and experienced professionals who will provide a higher standard of care for imaging patients.

The encouragement of diversity requires individuals to move beyond the Western tradition by broadening their learning and opening their minds to new forms of thought.[5] As teachers mentor students through the educational process, they also must assist them in moving beyond any self-centered worldviews. Even students from similar geographic locations and of similar races bring unique insights to the class as a result of their differing experiences and backgrounds. As they share these differences, they increase their knowledge base, which provides them with greater empathy for their patients and one another. This intellectual broadening is a crucial component in establishing an appropriate educational and working environment for people of many backgrounds.

MULTICULTURALISM
Multiculturalism is respect for the diversity of the many ways of knowing beyond the Western model, brought about by a broadening of learning and an opening of the mind to new ways of thought.

Adaptation of resources for people of all backgrounds is termed *multiculturalism*. All the variables identified in issues relating to diversity also must be considered in discussions of multiculturalism.

Interaction Patterns

-ISMs
-isms are prejudgments entailing a tendency to judge others according to a standard considered ideal or presumed to be "normal."

Imaging professionals should be able to recognize the interaction patterns commonly encountered when issues of diversity are discussed. These interaction patterns are labeled *-isms* because of their common word endings. Each -ism involves a tendency to judge others according to a standard considered ideal or presumed to be "normal." They are grounded in bias, prejudicial in attitude, and discriminatory in their behavioral expression. An -ism is centered on personal judgment, regardless of evidence (Box 8-1).[6]

BOX 8-1 THE -ISMs

ableism The assumption that people who are able-bodied and sound of mind are physically or developmentally superior to those who are physically or developmentally disabled or otherwise different. Ableism occurs when medical professionals do not offer choices to patients who are chronically ill because they assume such patients do not want to or cannot make decisions.

adultism The assumption that adults are superior to youths and can or should control, direct, reprimand, and reward them or deprive them of respect. Children in American society often are interrupted or ignored by adults. They may not be given choices that allow them to feel they have some control over a situation.

ageism The assumption that members of one age group are superior to those of others. Young patients and staff members may not be taken as seriously as those who are older; in other circumstances, older persons may be discredited in favor of those who are younger.

classism, or elitism The assumption that certain people are superior because of their social status, economic status, or position in a group or organization. This prejudgment assumes that those with more money or education are superior to people lacking in money or formal schooling. Elitism may occur in medicine if a poorly dressed high school dropout is not given the same treatment options offered to a well-dressed college graduate.

egocentrism The assumption that oneself is superior to others. Egocentrism has occurred if a person (e.g., a staff member) who has never been diagnosed with a mental illness feels superior to a patient with a mental illness.

BOX 8-1 THE -ISMs—cont'd

ethnocentrism The assumption that one's own cultural or ethnic group is superior to that of others. (*Ethnicity* refers to cultural differences other than race.) An organization or country may be ethnocentric if it expects all persons regardless of country of origin to speak a certain language or know a set of implicit rules for conduct that may be peculiar to that organization or country.

heterosexism The assumption that everyone is, or should be, heterosexual and that heterosexuality is superior and expectable. Only recently was homosexuality redefined as a lifestyle rather than a disease.

racism The assumption that members of one race are superior to those of another. (*Race* refers to presumed biologic differences based on skin color.)

sexism The assumption that members of one gender are superior to those of the other. For example, women have historically been viewed as being less rational and more emotional than men.

sizism The assumption that people of one body size are superior to or better than those of other shapes and sizes. Positions involving interaction with the public, for example, may be denied to individuals who are very heavy or otherwise fail to meet arbitrary standards of ideal appearance.

sociocentrism The assumption that one society's intellectual methods or actions are superior to the ways of other societies. For instances, Western medical practitioners may feel that biomedicine is effective and folk medicines are not, even when strong evidence exists that this is not always the case. Many traditional societies have highly effective, community-oriented forms of treatment.

IMAGING SCENARIO

An imaging student from an affluent background is assigned to a clinical rotation providing chest radiographs in an urban medical center. The center provides care to many indigent and homeless people who require imaging services. The student has a great deal of difficulty understanding why these patients are unable to provide homes for themselves and why they are not employed. This lack of understanding affects the student's ability to communicate with patients and project the caring attitude that is essential to quality imaging services. After clinical grades have been given for this rotation, the student is dismayed to receive a much lower score than he anticipated. He approaches his instructor and questions the grade.

Discusion questions

- What issues might the instructor discuss with the student?
- In what way do these issues affect ethical problem solving for this student?
- Can the student's attitudes and perceptions be remedied? Should they be?

A Study in Diversity

A study was conducted in a Midwestern state concerning the incorporation of diversity topics into the imaging sciences curriculum.[7] Researchers gathered information with a survey that asked a variety of questions of the program's directors and students. The majority of respondents answered that topics relating to diversity were important and should be included in the curriculum. A sampling of the comments provided in answer to the survey that may be of interest to imaging professionals is included in Boxes 8-2 and 8-3. A small percentage of students enrolled in the programs believed that issues of multiculturalism and diversity are not important to the imaging curriculum. The researcher was concerned by this result. If students do not believe that an understanding of the differences among patients is important, patient care may suffer. Students who do not support multiculturalism may hold that all patients should be treated equally and medicine should be color-blind or blind to other differences. This implies that all patients have the same needs or that all patients should be treated with equal quality of service. Imaging students would do well to remember that patients are unique and deserve imaging professionals able to recognize individual needs, but they do also all deserve quality imaging services. Program directors need to investigate issues of diversity early in the educational program. Caring requires an identification with and respect for the needs of all patients. When students respect differences, they are better able to care for patients.

BOX 8-2 PROGRAM DIRECTORS' UNEDITED INDIVIDUAL COMMENTS

- We are beginning to explore these issues and how to integrate them into the curriculum.
- JCAHO [Joint Commission on Accreditation of Healthcare Organizations] requirements include in-service education involving diversity.
- ASRT educators' group listed diversity issues as important to core curriculum development.
- I believe that if you would add this topic as a part of the curriculum, it would be important to have the class at the start of the first year.
- Multiculturalism and diversity could be interlaced into current patient care classes.
- In patient care there is some discussion about language barriers, age and ability problems. Also, there are some ethics discussion dealing with sexuality, race and religion, but no actual unit on cultural differences.
- I agree that multiculturalism and diversity should be included within the program, but may be added to an already existing class.
- We do very little and should do more on this subject. I don't think we have the time to include an entire course but guest lecturers from other cultures would be beneficial. I may incorporate this into our class.

From Towsley D: Assessing the skill requirements for radiographers in the traditional and patient-focused care settings, *Radiol Sci Educ* 2(1): , 1995.

BOX 8-3 STUDENTS' UNEDITED INDIVIDUAL COMMENTS

- A lot of people don't handle working with diverse people. People have been brought up to stay with their own kind of people, but today people need to learn to interact with different people.
- I think everyone should learn more about how to communicate with different people. I know it would help me.
- Everyone who works in the hospital needs to have a working knowledge of the different cultures. It would be a good idea to teach some beginning Spanish classes as we are in contact with many Hispanics that speak no or little English.
- Since you deal with a variety of people you should be educated about them.
- I believe everyone is different and has different needs. I do the best I can to meet these needs while producing the best possible x-ray.
- I think this is important for people to be multiculturally educated, but it should be in your heart to treat people as if they were all the same.
- I think overall patients have the same basic needs—but learning about specific cultures would be helpful to make the specific patient feel more comfortable.
- Throughout my life I have personally went out to get to know other cultures and I enjoy them so much. But a lot of students maybe have not and I think it would be beneficial to have multicultural education. We need to know some cultural differences to help us communicate with patients better.
- I'm not sure how multiculturalism and diversity relate to radiography except the fact that each radiographer should be able to relate to each patient effectively no matter what the race is. The family style, ability, appearance, etc. really shouldn't matter to the radiographer. Treat each patient equally. We should be informed of the diversity in the radiography field. I agree with that 100 percent.
- Some everyday actions to us can be insulting to people of different cultures. It would be helpful to know these.
- It would probably be beneficial if more staff technologists or students had a basic knowledge of other languages, especially Spanish. This being the more common one that I've run into, there is a definite barrier there if there's no communication—perhaps the hospital needs more interpreters or availability.
- I think multiculturalism issues are important since patients are all unique and as we are placed in other areas of the United States we will be impacted by this. As a student who took classes that dealt with diversity and its issues, I have found much of this knowledge to be more useful than I expected. This is why I think multiculturalism is an important part of all education.
- I think a course dealing with multiculturalism would be very useful in helping both to educate and break down barriers between cultures. Some multicultural education is needed.

Program directors and students should be encouraged to become active in encouraging the incorporation of diversity into the curriculum to enhance patient care and make imaging professionals more sensitive to the needs of others. Sensitivity to the differences among individuals allows imaging professionals to understand better patients' differing reactions to the imaging environment, the way patients make choices, and the need to employ ethical decision making. It also allows them to identify a variety of methods to explain imaging procedures to a diverse patient population. These methods may include language courses, visual aids, interpreters, patient advocates, and informational sessions presented as continuing education by a variety of presenters.

Imaging professionals should consider issues of diversity before performing imaging procedures to facilitate a more comfortable environment for communication between them and their patients. They must recognize their responsibility to adapt to the needs of patients from all backgrounds.

DIVERSITY AND ETHICS

Many ethical issues are involved in dealing with a diverse patient population. By recognizing, accepting, and learning ways to accommodate this diversity, imaging professionals become much more adept at providing care that protects patient autonomy, right to information (informed consent process), and confidentiality.

The ages and mental abilities of patients often have an impact on the ethical challenges faced by imaging professionals. For example, an elderly patient with Alzheimer's disease scheduled to have a barium enema is most likely unable to have a truly informed consent process. Such a patient may require an advocate.

IMAGING SCENARIO

A small child arrives in the radiography department to have an intravenous pyelogram (IVP). The child has been raised in a home in which only German is spoken; the child is not of school age and speaks no English. The parent tells the child to behave and leaves the room. Now the radiographer and radiologist, neither of whom speak German, have to try to help this child understand the procedure and aid him in tolerating it.

Discussion questions

- Why would the parent leave the child?
- What are the differences in what is expected of children growing up in this culture?
- In what ways could the imaging professionals have been better prepared to protect the child and make this procedure less traumatic?
- What are some practical approaches to this situation?

Truthfulness and confidentiality also enter into some diversity challenges. In some cultures the elders of the family make decisions for all family members. This hierarchy may affect the radiologist who is explaining the procedure and discussing alternatives to treatment. Confidentiality may be diminished or lost in situations in which patients are having life decisions made for them by others but need to share information they do not wish the rest of the family to know with the radiologist.

Many situations require knowledge of the similarities and differences in patients and cultures. The more imaging professionals know about diversity, the more they can ready themselves for these interactions. Certain acceptable approaches are recommended for interactions of imaging professionals with all cultural groups (Box 8-4). In addition, categories for basic cultural assessment enable imaging professionals to provide quality imaging services for a variety of patients (Box 8-5).

BOX 8-4 APPROACHES RECOMMENDED FOR ALL CULTURAL GROUPS

- Provide a feeling of acceptance.
- Establish open communication.
- Present yourself with confidence. Introduce yourself. Shake hands if appropriate.
- Strive to gain your patient's trust, but do not be resentful if you do not receive it.
- Understand what "caring" means to members of the cultural or subcultural group, both attitudinally and behaviorally.
- Understand the relationship between your patient and authority.
- Understand patients' desire to please you and their motivations to comply.
- Anticipate diversity. Avoid stereotypes by gender, age, ethnicity, or socioeconomic status.
- Do not make assumptions about where people come from. Let them tell you.
- Understand the patient's goals and expectations.
- Make your own goals realistic.
- Emphasize positive points and strengths of minority health beliefs and practices.
- Show respect to all family members present, especially to men, even if the patient is a woman or child. Men often are decision makers regarding follow-up care.
- Be prepared for the fact that children go everywhere with parents in some cultural groups and in poorer families, who may have few child care options. Include them.
- Know the traditional health-related practices common to the group with which you are working. Do not discredit them unless you *know* they are harmful.
- Know the folk illnesses and remedies common to the group with which you are working.
- Try to make the clinic setting comfortable. Consider colors, music, atmosphere, scheduling expectations, pace, and seating arrangements.
- Whenever possible and appropriate, involve the leaders of the local group.
- Confidentiality is important, but community leaders know local problems and often can suggest acceptable interventions.
- Respect values, beliefs, rights, and practices. Some may come into conflict with your own values or your determination to make changes. Nevertheless, every group and individual deserves to be treated with respect.
- Learn to appreciate the richness of diversity as an asset rather than a hindrance in your work.

BOX 8-5 CATEGORIES FOR A BASIC CULTURAL ASSESSMENT

- Ethnic origin, identity, affiliation, values (ideas about health and illness, human nature, relationships between humankind and nature, time, activity, and interpersonal relationships), relevant rites of passage, customs, art and symbols, and history
- Racial identity (ask, do not assume)
- Place of birth; relocation and migration history
- Habits, customs, and beliefs associated with health, disease, illness, health maintenance, illness prevention, and health promotion; explanatory models; connections between health and religion
- Cultural sanctions and restrictions (behaviors that are encouraged or discouraged)
- Language and communication processes (verbal and nonverbal patterns, eye contact, use of and toleration for touching, silence, tempo, styles of questioning and persuasion, styles of decision making)
- Gender rules
- Healing beliefs and practices (relationships with folk, popular, and professional health systems; symbolism related to health and illness; behaviors that are considered normal or abnormal; care associated with unusual or abnormal behavior; care associated with body fluids, excretions and secretions, and temperature; activities included in tending to one's body; substances and practices used in rituals; myths about health; taboos [substances and events to be avoided]; and ideas and practices related to death, dying, and grief)
- Nutritional factors; food preferences, preparation, and consumption patterns (kinds of foods and amounts, schedules and rituals, eating environments, utensils and implements, taboos, changes with illness)
- Sleep routines, bedtime rituals, and environment (kinds of covering, sleepwear, comforting materials used, rules for sleeping and awakening)
- Environmental resources and strains (the "fit" within the community)
- Economic status, resources, and living situation
- Educational history and background
- Occupational history and background
- Social network (types and amount of support available from family, other individuals, and group resources; who and where extended family and significant others are; what is expected and expectable from them; social interaction patterns)
- Self-identity or self-concept and sense of well-being
- Religious history, background, and beliefs
- Other spiritual beliefs and practices
- Usual response to stress and discomfort
- Meaning of care and caring (expectations, beliefs, and practices related to care; relationships between providers and patients as cultural seekers of health care and between patients and the health care system)

VALUES AND DIVERSITY

So far this chapter has discussed the importance of respecting the ways in which human beings differ from one another, but imaging professionals also should realize that individuals are more alike than they are different. Every group and individual must manage the same basic requirements of living to survive and thrive; to do so, they choose and follow a set of values. These universal values include orientation toward nature (including the supernatural), time, activity, relationships with other people, and the nature of humankind.[8] Imaging professionals should understand their place and that of the patient in the continua of values (see Figure 1-1). They also should consider the ways in which others' worldviews differ from their own. This consideration enables imaging professionals to understand themselves, their colleagues, and their patients better and in doing so become more effective in recognizing their own and others' perspectives and the ways in which they influence relationships.[3]

Imaging professionals must be able to understand their patients' values and worldviews. Ethical decision making requires an acceptance that human beings share values and worldviews, often in spite of other differences. This realization provides a foundation for empathy and truly ethical problem solving.

LEGAL ISSUES

A consideration of discrimination laws is vital in any legal discussion of diversity issues. Many state and federal laws prohibit discrimination on the basis of race, gender, age, national origin, religion, or disability. These laws have a profound impact on the imaging professional in both employment and patient treatment situations.

The federal statutes most commonly invoked in prohibiting discrimination in employment situations include Title VII of the Civil Rights Act of 1964,[9] the Equal Pay Act of 1964,[10] the Age Discrimination in Employment Act (ADEA) of 1967,[11] the Rehabilitation Act of 1973,[12] the Americans with Disabilities Act (ADA) of 1990,[13] and the Family and Medical Leave Act of 1993.[14] The federal statutes most commonly invoked in prohibiting discrimination in patient treatment include the Emergency Medical Treatment and Labor Act,[15] Title VI of the 1964 Civil Rights Act,[16] Section 504 of the Rehabilitation Act of 1974,[17] and the Americans with Disabilities Act.[18]

Many of these antidiscrimination statutes are examined in this chapter in the context of employment and patient treatment discrimination. State antidiscrimination statutes also often come into play, but because they are diverse and generally similar to federal statutes, they are not examined here.

ANTIDISCRIMINATION STATUTES IN EMPLOYMENT SITUATIONS

Title VII of the Civil Rights Act of 1964[9] prohibits discrimination because of race, color, gender, religion, or national origin. This is the most commonly used statute in employment discrimination cases; it prohibits both discipline and discharge based on any of the reasons previously stated and also prohibits any employer from retaliating against an employee exercising any of these protected rights.

The Equal Pay Act of 1964[10] prohibits discrimination based on gender. It also requires equal compensation for equal work on jobs requiring equal skill, effort, and responsibility when performed under similar working conditions.

The ADEA[11] prohibits discrimination based on age. It protects employees ages 40 and older from discrimination in employment—including discharge based on age—and applies both to private and public employees.

The Rehabilitation Act of 1973[12] and the ADA[13] both protect employees from discrimination based on disability. The Rehabilitation Act applies to federal employers and some private employers performing work for the federal government. The ADA's prohibition of discrimination based on disability is broader than that of the Rehabilitation Act and includes disabled status, perception of disability, or a record of physical or mental impairment. The ADA applies to private employers but specifically excludes the U.S. government. Under the ADA, employers must provide equal employment opportunities for disabled employees by making reasonable accommodations.

The Family and Medical Leave Act of 1993[14] applies to private employers who have 50 or more employees. It also applies to employees who have been employed for 1 year or longer. It allows employees to take as much as 12 weeks unpaid leave during any 12-month period for a number of reasons:

- To give birth to a child and provide care for the infant
- To care for a spouse, parent, or child with a serious health condition
- To recover from a serious health condition that prevents the employee from properly performing the job

The Act also prohibits employers from discriminating against employees who use such leave and provides for an equivalent position, pay, and other terms and conditions of employment after such leave.

Although each of these laws is complex, some general elements may be extracted to provide a working framework of employment discrimination law. The following paragraphs discuss employment discrimination cases in general, sexual harassment cases more specifically, and the legal guidelines that must be followed in the workplace.

Employment Discrimination

Employment discrimination claims are based on statutes. These statutes provide procedures for enforcement of the statutes and time restrictions for filing claims. These procedures must be followed to obtain relief based on these statutes. Many states also allow for private lawsuits, but the filing of a complaint with the appropriate agency is generally a prerequisite to a private cause of action, as is filing a timely complaint with the state's enforcement agency (such as the Civil Rights Commission).

Many employment discrimination cases involve situations in which employees feel they have been treated differently than other similarly employed individuals. These are called *disparate treatment cases.* Employment discrimination also may be claimed if the policies of an employer have an unfair impact on employees who belong to protected groups (such as women). These are called *disparate impact cases.* Employment discrimination also includes retaliatory actions by employers against employees who exercise their rights under antidiscrimination statutes. Guidance on such cases was established in the landmark 1973 United States Supreme Court case of *McDonnell Douglas v Green*[19] and clarified through many other cases.

McDonnell Douglas[19] established that to make a claim of employment discrimination, the employee must first establish a prima facie case. This means that the employee, or complainant, must first show that the following conditions have been met:

1. The complainant belongs to a protected class (e.g., woman, ethnic or racial minority, disabled).
2. The complainant was qualified for the position.
3. Despite the qualifications, the complainant was not hired or was discharged.
4. The employer continued to look for an individual with the complainant's qualifications to fill the position or hired an individual less qualified than the complainant who was not a member of that protected class.

The establishment of a prima facie case does not prove the complainant was a victim of discrimination. It does, however, establish the proper foundation for the employee to file a claim with the appropriate enforcement agency, such as the Equal Employment Opportunity Commission (EEOC).

PRIMA FACIE CASE OF EMPLOYMENT DISCRIMINATION
A prima facie case of employment discrimination is what must be proved by a complainant making a claim of employment discrimination. It requires complainants to prove they belong to a protected class, were qualified for the position, were not hired or were discharged, and after their discharge the employer continued to look for an individual with the complainant's qualifications to fill the position or hired an individual less qualified than the complainant who was not a member of that protected class.

Sexual Harassment

Case law has consistently interpreted the prohibition of gender discrimination in Title VII to include the forbidding of sexual harassment on the job. Because sexual harassment claims are the most frequent employment discrimination claims, imaging professionals will benefit from an understanding of the applicable laws.

The EEOC[21] has established guidelines defining sexual harassment, which the court has recognized:

> Harassment on the basis of sex is a violation of Section 703 of Title VII. Unwelcome sexual advances, requests for sexual favors, and other verbal and physical conduct of a sexual nature constitute sexual harassment when (1) submission to such conduct is made either explicitly or implicitly a term or condition of an individual's employment, (2) submission to or rejection of such conduct by an individual is used as the basis for employment decisions affecting such individual, or (3) such conduct has the purpose or effect of unreasonably interfering with an individual's work performance or creating an intimidating, hostile, or offensive working environment.

SEXUAL HARASSMENT
Sexual harassment includes unwelcome sexual advances, requests for sexual favors, and other verbal and physical conduct of a sexual nature that the employee is required to submit to as a term or condition of employment; submission to, or rejection of, such conduct is used as the basis for employment decisions; or such conduct has the purpose or effect of unreasonably interfering with an individual's work performance or creating an intimidating, hostile, or offensive working environment.

Two types of sexual harassment claims have been recognized by the courts under these guidelines. They are quid pro quo and hostile work environment claims.

Quid pro quo claims assert that initial or continued employment or advancement depends on sexual conduct. A supervisor or manager must necessarily be involved in quid pro quo sexual harassment cases.[20]

Hostile work environment claims argue that the harassment unreasonably interferes with the employee's work performance or creates an intimidating, hostile, or offensive work environment. These cases usually involve conduct such as sexual

QUID PRO QUO SEXUAL HARASSMENT
Quid pro quo sexual harassment occurs when initial or continued employment or advancement depends on sexual conduct. A supervisor or manager must necessarily be involved in quid pro quo sexual harassment cases.

HOSTILE WORK ENVIRONMENT SEXUAL HARASSMENT
Hostile work environment sexual harassment occurs when sexual behaviors unreasonably interfere with work performance or create an intimidating, hostile, or offensive work environment. Sexual suggestions, sexually derogatory remarks, and sexually motivated physical contact may constitute hostile work environment sexual harassment. Actions of supervisors, co-workers, and customers can give rise to hostile work environment claims. Employers are liable if they create or condone a discriminatory work environment.

suggestions, sexually derogatory remarks, and sexually motivated physical contact. Early cases required a finding that the harassment was so severe it seriously affected the employee's psychologic well-being.[20] However, more recent cases have held that if a reasonable person would find the working environment hostile or abusive and the victim perceives the environment to be abusive, a hostile work environment may be found.[22] The loss of tangible job benefits is not a prerequisite to a hostile work environment claim.[23] Actions of supervisors, co-workers, and customers can give rise to hostile work environment claims. Employers are liable if they create or condone a discriminatory work environment.[23]

IMAGING SCENARIO

A male technologist is hired to perform computed tomography (CT) by the female director of radiology. The director, as early as the interview, hints to the applicant that she is romantically available and thinks he is attractive. Throughout his first few months of employment, the director pays special attention to him and continues to hint at her availability. The technologist lets the director know that he is currently seeing someone, and even introduces his significant other to the director when she comes to meet him for lunch.

Over the next year, the director continues to pay special attention to the technologist, makes comments about his attractiveness, and even states that she would like to get together with him. The technologist laughs off these comments as best he can. The position of supervisor of CT opens. The director approaches the male technologist and informs him that the position is his if he will become intimate with her.

- Is this sexual harassment?
- What kind of harassment is this?
- Is the hospital liable for the acts of the director? What can the technologist do?

Discussion

This is quid pro quo sexual harassment. It is quid pro quo because the advancement of the technologist depends on sexual conduct and the demand is made by his supervisor. Because this is quid pro quo, the employer will be liable for the conduct of its supervisors, whether or not they were aware of the conduct, even if the conduct was not authorized or was forbidden. There should be a policy within the facility for the technologist to address the harassment internally. The technologist has a right to file a complaint with the Civil Rights Commission and the EEOC. After compliance with the Civil Rights Commission and EEOC procedures, the technologist could file a lawsuit against the director and the facility.

Prima Facie Hostile Work Environment

To make a claim for hostile work environment sexual harassment, the complainant must first establish a prima facie case[22, 24]:

1. The employee must be a member of a protected class.
2. The employee must have been subject to unwelcome sexual harassment in the form of sexual advances, requests for sexual favors, or other verbal or physical conduct of a sexual nature.
3. The complaint of harassment must have been based on gender.
4. The alleged sexual harassment must have had the effect of unreasonably interfering with the employee's work performance and creating a working environment a reasonable person would find intimidating, hostile, abusive, or offensive and the employee perceived as abusive.
5. The employer knew or should have known of the harassment and failed to take appropriate action.

Whether the alleged misconduct is severe enough to be considered hostile or abusive and thus resulting in liability is a question to be determined in light of all the circumstances of the employment relationship.[24] Case law has held that the mere presence of an employee who has engaged in particularly severe or pervasive sexual harassment may create a hostile work environment. EEOC guidelines[25] require investigation of the nature of the sexual advances and the context in which the alleged misconduct occurred; the legality of the actions is determined on a case-by-case basis.[26]

Who is Protected?

Both men and women are protected by sexual harassment statutes, and harassing conduct toward homosexual and heterosexual individuals is prohibited. However, harassment arising because of a person's sexual preference is not protected under sexual harassment statutes because it is not based on gender.[27] For example, a prima facie case was not established by a male employee who was forced to resign because his co-workers did not approve of his relationship with another man.[27] However, Title VII does protect employees from harassment resulting from terminated consensual relationships.[28] An employer may be liable for sex discrimination if employment opportunities or benefits are granted because of an employee's submission to sexual advances or requests. Qualified employees who were denied opportunities because of their refusal to grant sexual favors may have a sexual harassment claim.[29]

What Is Unwelcome?

Conduct must be unwanted and offensive to be prohibited under Title VII. As stated previously, the determination of whether conduct is sufficiently hostile or abusive to be actionable must be determined in the light of all the circumstances of the employment relationship.[22, 24]

Generally courts must find that the complainant made some effort to indicate that the conduct was unwelcome or offensive. In one case, a court found that because a workplace was one in which sexual horseplay was consensual and the complainant participated in telling sexual jokes, the complainant was not offended to the point of sexual harassment by a sexually explicit cartoon given to her by her supervisor.[30]

Another court found that a personnel director's close attention to a complainant was not unwelcome harassment because the complainant had been giving the personnel director mixed signals by sharing many personal problems with him. Additionally, her requests for him to leave her alone were not delivered with any sense of emergency, sincerity, or force.[31] Yet another court found that conduct in a female-run quality-control shop in which sexual innuendo and vulgarity were commonplace and both male and female employees, including the plaintiff, took part in such conduct did not give rise to a Title VII sexual harassment action.[32]

When Are Employers Liable?

Generally, employers are liable for any quid pro quo sexual harassment committed by their supervisory personnel, even if the conduct was not authorized or was even forbidden.[24] This is generally true regardless of whether the employer knew or should have known of the conduct.[33]

In hostile work environment cases, employer liability is not as clear. Most courts have imposed liability if the employer knew or should have known that a supervisor's behavior created a hostile work environment and failed to take prompt remedial action.[24]

Harassment in the workplace by co-workers also may create liability for the employer if the employer or supervisory personnel knew or should have known of the harassing behavior and failed to respond promptly and in a manner likely to prevent recurrent behavior.[33] Employers are generally found liable only if the alleged offensive conduct is severe and pervasive and not if the offensive conduct is sporadic or occurs in isolated incidents.[22]

EEOC guidelines[21] provide direction for employers in preventing sexual harassment. After employers become aware of potential sexual harassment, they must take prompt and adequate remedial action. The EEOC encourages prevention of sexual harassment in the workplace[21]:

> An employer should take all steps necessary to prevent sexual harassment from occurring, such as affirmatively raising the subject, expressing strong disapproval, developing appropriate sanctions, informing employees of their right to raise and how to raise the issue of harassment under Title VII, and developing methods to sensitize all concerned.

Health care facilities should have policies to inform employees of conduct constituting sexual harassment, express disapproval of such conduct, facilitate the handling of sexual harassment complaints, clearly identify procedures for dealing with such complaints, describe the manner in which they will be investigated, and list the sanctions to be expected for harassing behavior. Procedures should be fair both to complainant and accused.

The health care facility's policies and procedures should clearly specify to whom reports of sexual harassment should be made and the correct procedure to be followed. A person who feels sexually harassed has a right to file a complaint with the Civil Rights Commission and the EEOC. There are time limitations for filing these complaints, which were discussed earlier. After complying with the Civil Rights Commission and the EEOC procedures, the plaintiff may file a lawsuit against the facility.

Imaging departments in most health care facilities provide opportunities for close work with many individuals, including physicians, nurses, other imaging professionals, students, and patients. Imaging professionals must be aware of conduct constituting sexual harassment and their rights and obligations if such behavior occurs, including the duty to state clearly that the conduct is offensive and unwelcome. They also should work to prevent allegations of sexual harassment by avoiding taking part in sexual jokes, teasing, innuendo, and other situations that may be misinterpreted by others.

IMAGING SCENARIO

A female technologist is hired just after graduation at a hospital across town from where she trained. This hospital does a great deal of orthopedic work, and the majority of her time is to be spent taking radiographs in surgery. The first day she is shocked by the language used in the surgical suite and the subject matter of the discussions. She soon realizes that it is normal procedure for the physicians and surgery staff to tell off-color jokes about sex and even to discuss each other's sexual adventures. She is embarrassed by this behavior but says nothing. Within a few weeks, they start teasing her about her sexual behavior and making sexual suggestions to her. She complains to her supervisor. Her supervisor visits with the surgery supervisor, who brushes the behavior off as insignificant. Within a few months, the technologist dreads going to work and has even called in sick several times just to avoid the situation.

- Is this sexual harassment?
- What kind of harassment is this?
- Is the hospital liable for these acts?
- What can the technologist do?

Discussion

This is hostile work environment sexual harassment. The technologist is a member of a protected class, a woman. The determination as to whether the conduct is severe enough to be considered hostile or abusive and thus actionable must be determined in light of all the circumstances of the employment relationship. The technologist made some efforts to communicate that the conduct was offensive and unwelcome by complaining to her supervisor. Additionally, the technologist did not participate in the behavior. The fact that the technologist called in sick to avoid the situation also supports her

Continued

IMAGING SCENARIO—cont'd

claim that she perceived the environment as abusive or offensive and that it interfered with her work performance. Finally, the employer, through the technologist's supervisor and the surgery supervisor, knew or should have known of the harassment and failed to take appropriate action. Whether this behavior rises to an actionable level needs to be determined on a case-by-case basis in light of all the circumstances. The behavior leading to the complaint must be examined to determine whether a reasonable person would find the working environment hostile or abusive and whether the victim perceived it as hostile or abusive. Clearly the EEOC guidelines requiring an investigation into alleged sexual misconduct were not followed here. If the conduct is found to be severe enough to be actionable, the employer would likely be liable because it knew or should have known of the behavior and did not take prompt remedial action to prevent it.

A policy should be in place within the facility for the technologist to address the harassment internally. The technologist has a right to file a complaint with the Civil Rights Commission and the EEOC. After compliance with the Civil Rights Commission and EEOC procedures, the technologist could file a lawsuit against the facility.

ANTIDISCRIMINATION STATUTES IN PATIENT TREATMENT SITUATIONS

The Emergency Medical Treatment and Labor Act[15] (also called the Anti-Dumping Act) requires hospitals covered by its provisions to provide emergency medical screening examinations and treatment to stabilize serious medical conditions to all patients who come to the emergency department. Women in labor are to be delivered if inadequate time for transfer exists. The Act applies to all hospitals that participate in the federal Medicare program and have emergency departments.

Title VII of the 1964 Civil Rights Act[16] was passed to prevent discrimination against minorities in federally funded programs. The statute provides that "No person in the United States shall on the ground of race, color, or national origin, be excluded from participation in, be denied the benefits of, or be subjected to discrimination under any program or activity receiving Federal financial assistance." Most hospitals, nursing homes, and health care institutions receive federal funds and therefore must comply with the antidiscrimination provisions of Title VII.

Section 504 of the Rehabilitation Act of 1974[17] and the ADA[13] prohibit discrimination against persons who are disabled. The Rehabilitation Act applies only to facilities receiving federal funds. The ADA, however, applies to public accommodations operated by private entities. Both Acts provide for private rights of action. The Department of Justice enforces the public accommodation provisions of the ADA.

Although technical differences between the two statutes exist, violations of one or both are generally alleged in claims of denial of treatment. Both include an exception to the duty to provide services if the disabled person presents a "direct threat" to the health and safety of others. *Direct threat* is defined as a significant risk that cannot be eliminated by a modification of policies, practices, or procedures, or by the provision of auxiliary aids or services.

The ADA[18] more explicitly addresses persons with human immunodeficiency virus (HIV) and acquired immunodeficiency syndrome (AIDS) and identifies more specific duties of providers; however, the ADA's suspension of such duties if a threat to others exists may limit its effectiveness. Some state legislatures have specifically made refusal to treat persons with AIDS illegal, and some statutes prohibiting discrimination against disabled persons may create an obligation to treat persons with AIDS and HIV. Physicians and other health care workers also have an ethical obligation to treat patients in need.

Imaging professionals are bound by the laws previously discussed. They also are bound by the ethical duty enumerated in Principle Three of the ASRT code of ethics[34] to "deliver patient care and service unrestricted by the concerns of physical attributes or the nature of the disease or illness, and without discrimination regardless of sex, race, creed, religion, or socioeconomic status."

OTHER DIVERSITY AND DISCRIMINATION ISSUES IN THE IMAGING PROFESSIONS

Males in Mammography

Although program requirements for diagnostic imaging professionals state that graduates will perform breast procedures competently, in reality this may be quite difficult for male students. They must be able to obtain the practical experience needed to reach proficiency in a procedure that most women are more comfortable having performed by a woman.

Conflicting values and legal obligations may exist in such situations. Facilities and imaging professionals must consider patient autonomy, dignity, and consent issues in regard to a female patient's desire to have a female mammographer. However, these issues must be balanced with the right of male mammographers not to suffer discrimination. This balancing is generally not easy, but it is possible. Having the female patient fill out a questionnaire before a face-to-face meeting with the male technologist may help avoid embarrassment for both and screen out women who have strong feelings against having male mammographers.

According to a survey of women's opinions of male mammographers, some of the problems associated with this issue may be minimized.[35] Although 83% of women said they prefer female technologists, only 31% said they would reschedule an examination with a female technologist if "a professional, competent and qualified male technologist" were assigned to perform the examination. The survey also indicated that male mammographers who are aware of women's preferences, sensitive to their concerns, and considerate of their reservations are more acceptable to their patients. Comments indicated that professional demeanor, patient rapport, and clinical competence may be more significant factors to some women than the gender of the technologist.

Unfortunately, this problem does not stop at the end of the training program. What happens if the only job available to a group of imaging graduates involves mammography and two applicants, a man and a woman, are seeking the position? Does the woman get the job automatically? Is this discriminatory treatment?

Females in Nuclear Medicine Technology

According to current literature, a trend exists for women to avoid pursuing studies that involve the physical sciences and lead to technology-intensive careers. Predictions indicate that by the year 2000, the supply of graduates from nuclear medicine technology (NMT) schools will meet only 45% of the projected demand for employees. As a partial solution to this problem, NMT programs need to attract an increased number of female students.

The perception of gender bias influences the number of women who graduate from science- and technology-oriented educational programs. The creation of a gender-fair learning environment may help eliminate this perception. Much research has been done to explore the modifications necessary in curriculum, teaching techniques, and teacher behaviors necessary to create gender equality. One must wonder whether such increased efforts to recruit women into NMT programs may have a discriminatory effect on male applicants.

SUMMARY

Diversity has many definitions. Differences among individuals are rooted in culture, age, experience, health, gender, sexual orientation, race and ethnic identity, mental abilities, income, marital status, education, religion, and sociocultural status. Students must recognize their own uniqueness to appreciate that of others. They should avoid perpetuating "-isms"—interaction patterns that involve a tendency to judge others according to their correlation with a standard considered ideal or "normal."

Program directors and students who recognize the positive impact of making diversity a part of the curriculum need to be encouraged to include these topics in education so that patient care will be enhanced and students will become more sensitive to the needs of others. By recognizing, accepting, and learning ways to deal with diversity, imaging professionals become much more adept at providing care that protects patient autonomy, rights to information, informed consent processes, rights to the truth, and confidentiality.

Imaging professionals also should become aware of the similarities among all people. These similarities may be found in patients' value systems and worldviews; they provide a foundation for empathy and the realization that the need for ethical problem solving is universal.

An understanding of discrimination law is vital in legal discussions of diversity issues. Federal and state statutes prohibit discrimination on the basis of race, gender, age, national origin, religion, and disability. Codes of ethics also prohibit discrimination by health care workers, including imaging professionals. Discrimination is prohibited both in employment and in patient treatment situations. Statutes prohibiting discrimination in employment include Title VII of the Civil Rights Act of 1964, the Equal Pay Act, the ADEA, the Rehabilitation Act of 1973, the ADA, and the Family and Medical Leave Act.

Employment discrimination may be claimed if an employee is treated differently than a similarly employed individual because of a protected condition (e.g., race, gender, national origin, religion, disability). These are called *disparate treatment cases.* Employment discrimination also may be claimed if a policy has an unfair impact on a protected group. These are called *disparate impact cases.* Employment discrimination cases are investigated by the EEOC at the federal level and the Civil Rights Commission at the state level. Time limits for filing claims are rigorously enforced.

To file a discrimination claim, complainants must establish a prima facie case in which they prove membership in a protected group and qualification for the position, argue that despite qualification, they were not hired or were discharged, and note the employer continued to look for an individual with similar qualifications to fill the position or hired a less qualified individual who was not a member of the protected class.

Sexual harassment claims under Title VII are the most frequent employment discrimination claims made. The EEOC has established guidelines for behavior in the workplace, and case law has further defined these guidelines. Generally, two types of sexual harassment have been recognized—quid pro quo and hostile work environment. Quid pro quo harassment occurs if a supervisor requests sexual favors in return for continued employment or employment advancement. Hostile work environment harassment occurs if the sexually related conduct unreasonably interferes with the employee's work performance or creates an intimidating, hostile, or offensive work environment. The establishment of a prima facie hostile work environment claim requires the complainant to meet five specific conditions.

Whether the complained of conduct is unwelcome or severe enough to be considered hostile or abusive is determined in light of all the circumstances of the situation, on a case-by-case basis. Employers are liable for the actions of their supervisors in quid pro quo harassment cases. Employers are generally liable for harassment in the workplace if they or their supervisors knew or should have known of the harassment and failed to take immediate and appropriate corrective action.

A variety of statutes prohibit discrimination in patient care situations. In addition, the Emergency Medical Treatment and Labor Act requires hospitals that participate in the Medicare program and have emergency rooms to provide medical screening examinations and treatment to stabilize serious conditions to any patients entering the emergency department. Women in labor must be delivered if insufficient time for transfer exists.

Other statutes prohibit discrimination because of disability, HIV status, or AIDS. Exceptions to this prohibition may be made if the provision of services to the patient presents a direct threat to the health and safety of others. Nevertheless, imaging professionals have duties under these statutes and professional ethical guidelines to deliver patient care unrestricted by concerns of physical attributes or nature of illness and without discrimination regarding gender, creed, religion, or socioeconomic status.

Radiologic sciences provide other diversity issues, including the dilemma of male mammography technologists and the underrepresentation of women in NMT training programs. However, because issues of diversity are now better recognized, appropriate steps may be taken to minimize the problems related to them.

ENDNOTES

1. Spector RE: *Cultural diversity in health and illness,* ed 3, Norwalk, Conn., 1991, Appleton and Lange.
2. American Society of Radiologic Technologists National Education Consensus: *Radiography: the second century,* Albuquerque, NM, 1995, Author.
3. Kavanagh KH, Kennedy PH: *Promoting cultural diversity: strategies for health care professionals,* Newbury Park, Calif., 1992, Sage.
4. Hill-Storks H: *Dimensions of diversity,* American Health Care Radiology Administrators' 22nd Annual Meeting, Sudbury, Mass., 1994, American Health Care Radiology Administrators.
5. Marcus LR: Diversity and its discontents, *Review of Higher Education* 17:227, 1994.
6. Brislin R: *Understanding culture's influence on behavior,* Fort Worth, Tex., 1993, Harcourt Brace College.
7. Towsley DM: *The need for incorporating course work in cultural diversity in radiologic technology programs,* thesis, Cedar Falls, Ia., 1996, University of Northern Iowa.
8. Kluckhohn FR: Dominant and variant value orientations. In Kluckhohn C, Murray JA, editors: *Personality in nature, society and culture,* New York, 1971, Alfred A. Knopf.
9. 42 USCA Section 2000e et seq.
10. 29 USCA Sec 225.
11. 29 USCA Section 621 et seq.
12. 29 USCA Section 701 et seq.
13. 42 USCA Section 12-101 et seq.
14. Pub L 103-3.
15. 42 USCA Section 1395 (1994).
16. 42 USCA Section 2000 (1964).
17. 29 USCA Section 794.
18. 42 USCA Sections 12101-12213.
19. *McDonnell Douglas v Green,* 411 U.S. 792 (1973).
20. 29 CFR Section 1604.11 (a).
21. *Meritor Savings Bank v Vinson,* 106 S.Ct. 2399 (1986), citing other cases.
22. *Harris v Forklift Systems, Inc.,* 111 S.Ct. 367 (1993).
23. *Bundy v Jackson,* 641 F.2d 934 (D.C.Cir. 1981).
24. *Hensen v City of Dundee,* 682 F.2d.897 (11th Cir. 1982)
25. *Cline v General Electric Credit Auto Lease,* 784 F Supp. 650 (N.D. Ill. 1990).
26. 29 CFR Section 1604.11 (b).
27. *Carreno v IBEW Local No. 226,* 54 F.E.P. Cases 81 (D.Ka. 1990).
28. *William v Civiletti,* 487 F Supp. 1387 (D.D.C. 1980).
29. *Toscona v Nimmo,* 570 F Supp. 1197 (D. Del. 1983).
30. *Tindall v Housing Authority,* 762 F Supp. 259 (W.D. Ark. 1991).
31. *Kouri v Liberian Services,* 55 F.E.P. Cases 124, (E.D.Va. 1991).
32. *Wensheimer v Rockwell International Corp.,* 54 F.E.P. Cases 828 (M.D. Fla. 1990).
33. 29 CFR. 1604.11(d).
34. American Society of Radiologic Technologists and the American Registry of Radiologic Technologists: *Code of ethics,* Albuquerque, NM, 1994, Author.
35. Serbus C: Survey of women's opinions on male mammographers, *Radiol Technol* 65(3):174, 1994.

REVIEW QUESTIONS

1 Define *diversity.*
2 Define *multiculturalism.*
3 List the primary dimensions of diversity.
4 List the secondary dimensions of diversity.
5 ____________ ______________ are grounded in bias, prejudicial in attitude, and discriminatory in their behavioral expression.
6 What is the best time to provide educational opportunities in diversity issues for imaging students?
7 What does sensitivity to differences allow the imaging professional?
8 List three methods that might be employed to help patients from different cultures understand information about the examination.
9 Federal and state statutes prohibit discrimination on what basis?
10 Does anything besides the law prohibit discrimination by imaging professionals?
11 Title VII, the Equal Pay Act, the Age Discrimination in Employment Act, the Rehabilitation Act, and the Family and Medical Leave Act all prohibit discrimination in what area?
12 Employment discrimination in which an employee is treated differently from other similarly situated employees because of a protected condition is called ________________ ________________.
13 Employment discrimination in which a policy has a negative impact on a protected group is called ________________ ________________.
14 List the four conditions required for a prima facie case of employment discrimination.
15 What is the most frequent kind of employment discrimination claim brought under Title VII?
16 ____________________ ________________ ________________ harassment occurs if continued employment or advancement of employment depends on the provision of sexual favors.
17 ____________________ harassment occurs if the sexually related conduct unreasonably interferes with the employee's work performance or creates an intimidating, hostile, or offensive work environment.
18 List the five conditions required to establish a prima facie case of hostile work environment.
19 Imaging professionals have a legal and ethical duty to provide care to patients who are HIV-positive or have AIDS, with one exception. What is it?
20 **True or False** People are more alike than they are different.
21 **True or False** Diversity is only an issue of culture.
22 **True or False** Learning ways to accommodate diversity increases the patient's autonomy and confidentiality.
23 **True or False** The best time for the student to learn about diversity is at the end of the program.

24 **True or False** If a prima facie case of discrimination is established, the employee wins the case.

25 **True or False** Only the specific language or conduct that gave rise to the complaint is considered during the investigation of cases of sexual harassment.

26 **True or False** No duty exists for emergency departments to provide emergency treatment to patients without insurance.

CRITICAL THINKING QUESTIONS & ACTIVITIES

1 Discuss ways in which people are more alike than they are different.
2 Why is diversity important in imaging patient care? Justify your answer.
3 Analyze the ways in which uniqueness contributes to a better organization.
4 Select two -isms and explain the impact they have on imaging services.
5 Do you agree with the findings in the diversity study? Why or why not?
6 Describe educational methods to provide understanding of issues of diversity. Which are most likely to succeed?
7 Discuss the kind of conduct that may be interpreted as sexually harassing. Should you tell a sexually explicit (dirty) joke to your classmates? Should you tease fellow students about their sexual conduct? Should you date a fellow student?
8 Discuss the sexual discrimination policy in your facility. Do you know to whom you should report sexual harassment?
9 Discuss the male mammographer situation. Would a questionnaire truly help minimize embarrassment for patients unwilling to have a male mammographer perform their study? Would it help eliminate embarrassment for the male mammographer as well? Discuss the ways in which a male mammographer may help put a patient at ease.
10 Do female imaging professionals face similar situations? Discuss, for instance, female NMTs who must perform testicular scans. What techniques could female technologists use to help put patients at ease?
11 Prepare a scenario illustrating an ethical imaging challenge that diversity issues influence. Discuss the questions raised by the scenario.

PROFESSIONAL PROFILE

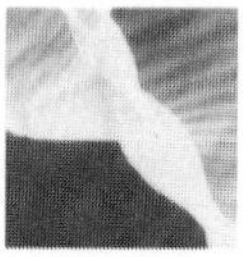

ETHICAL AND LEGAL ISSUES play important roles in an educator's position. It is extremely important that an educator stay abreast of specific legal ramifications related to the clinical aspect of patient care. It is also vital that this information be shared with students during orientation of the program and periodically throughout their educational endeavor.

I had a clinical experience that involved litigation and was not at all prepared to deal with a variety of issues. A student was helping a technologist with an erect shoulder radiograph of an elderly patient. The patient's daughter was in the room with the technologist, student, and patient. The patient was sitting on a rolling stool during the examination. After the radiographs were taken, the technologist informed both the student and the patient's relative to stay in the room with the patient while she went to check the films. As the technologist was entering the darkroom, she heard a loud noise, only to come and find the patient on the floor. The patient had suddenly moved and lost her balance on the rolling stool. This happened in front of both the student and the patient's relative. The technologist helped the patient onto the x-ray table. After a brief examination by the radiologist, a hip x-ray was taken. The patient had fractured her hip during the accident. At the time of the accident, the patient simply asked that her medical bills be paid, and no other demands were made. The patient was transferred to a local hospital and had surgical treatment of the fractured hip. On the patient's recovery, the patient's son (an attorney) came to visit the radiography clinic. He subpoenaed both the technologist and the student without anyone informing the faculty. Only after the fact was the faculty informed. At that time, the college appointed an attorney to investigate the case and stay abreast of the situation in case any litigation was necessary. One lesson learned from this was that it is not enough to just talk about these issues during orientation, but rather that it is necessary to continue discussing them throughout the 2 years.

In another case, a student x-rayed a patient who was pregnant. She shielded the patient and took necessary radiation protection precautions, but did so without consulting the staff technologist or radiologist. A written report was placed in the clinical files in case the patient decided to press litigation. The faculty learned once again to continue stressing the importance of ethical and legal issues to avoid litigation. A vital component of caring is following safety procedures.

MARTI MORENO, MS, RT(R), RDMS
CLINICAL COORDINATOR
RADIOGRAPHY PROGRAM
BLINN COLLEGE
Bryan, Texas

CHAPTER 9

Caring

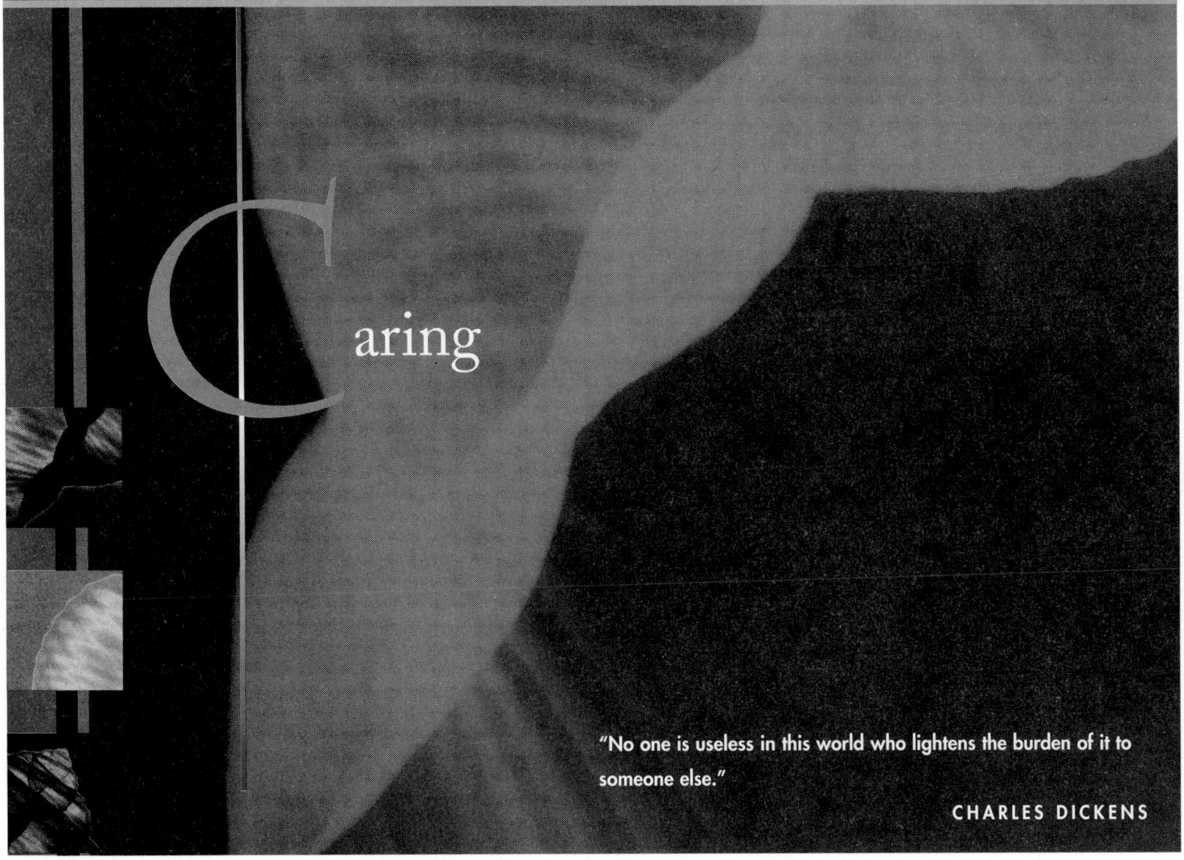

"No one is useless in this world who lightens the burden of it to someone else."

CHARLES DICKENS

LEARNING OBJECTIVES

- Understand the nature of care and its ethical and legal implications.
- Define *human care* and *professional care.*
- Understand care as a context for imaging practice.
- Discuss the development of a more caring demeanor.
- Explore the legal side of caring.

CHAPTER OUTLINE

ETHICAL ISSUES

Caring is essential for life and growth; it is a crucial ingredient in the imaging professional's ability to serve the needs of self and others. Caring requires the developmental strengths of trust, autonomy, initiative, identity, justice, industry, and intimacy, all of which play a role in discussions of ethics and ethical problem solving for the imaging professional.[1]

Health care professionals, including imaging professionals, refer to the therapy and other services they provide in their practices as *care.* Therefore caring is the primary task of the imaging professional. A caring attitude should influence the imaging professional's feelings and ethical problem solving arising from interactions with patients. This chapter defines caring, describes its ethical implications for imaging practice, and provides methods to help the imaging professional develop a more caring demeanor.

Eleanor McMartin has written "I Am the Patient," an essay illustrating a variety of issues discussed in this chapter (see page 168). This essay is a valuable reminder to imaging professionals of the important role they play in maintaining patient autonomy by projecting a caring attitude.

DEFINITION OF CARING

Caring is defined as a function in which a person expresses concern for the growth and well-being of another in an integrated application of the mind, body, and spirit designed to maximize positive outcomes. Expressions of caring include feelings of compassion and concern, a philosophy of commitment, an ethical approach to problems, altruistic acts, conscious attention to the needs and wishes of others, protection of well-being, nurturing of growth, and empathy and advocacy. Because it plays such a vital role in human interaction, an appreciation of caring is fundamental to an understanding of human nature.[2]

CARING
Caring is a function of the whole person in which concern for the growth and well-being of another is expressed in an integrated application of the mind, body, and spirit that seeks to maximize positive outcomes.

Activities such as listening, providing information, helping, communicating, and showing respect are expressions of caring.[3] Other caring activities include helping, touching, nurturing, supporting, and protecting (Box 9-1).[4] Caring is a universal phenomenon, although expressions, processes, and patterns may vary among cultures.[5]

BOX 9-1 EXPRESSIONS OF CARING

Advocacy	Courage
Altruism	Ethical behavior
Commitment	Monitoring
Compassion	Nurturing
Concern	Protection

EXISTENTIAL CARE
Existential care is compassion arising from an awareness of common bonds of humanity and common expressions, fates, and feelings.

Caring is essential in the development of the imaging professional.[6] Radiographers must be caring individuals, part scientist and part humanist. Humanism entails the provision of existential care, a more abstract form of care arising from an awareness of common bonds of humanity and common expressions, fates, and feelings.[7] Care may occur as a product of the rapport between imaging professionals and patients. Unfortunately, this is not always the case[8]:

> In radiology, particularly, the administrative focus is on reducing costs by increasing productivity. The efficiency of virtually every radiology department in this country is based on how many exams its technologists can complete per hour. This emphasis on speed means that radiologic technologists often must spend less time than they would like getting to know each patient. This can have a detrimental effect on patient satisfaction. Patients who are treated like bodies on a mechanized production line are bound to go somewhere else the next time they need health care. Patients who perceive a lack of genuine concern and empathy are the first to complain about their care and ask for their records to be transferred to another facility.

Care as an Ideal

Philosophically, care is an ideal analogous to beauty, truth, and justice; although it is sought after, it can never be fully attained or perfect in human expression.

IMAGING SCENARIO

A patient with a family history of breast cancer who has found a lump in her breast arrives at a mammography imaging center. She is frightened and emotional. She has read a great deal of literature about breast cancer and knows it is one of the leading causes of death in women. Her mother and sister died painful deaths at early ages, and she is frantic to learn her diagnosis. The breast imaging center has been informed that it needs to complete procedures more rapidly to allow a greater number of mammograms to be performed per day. This pressure for speed has elevated the stress of the mammographers. Moreover, unexpected emergencies and procedures that call for additional views cause backups in the waiting room, increasing the anxiety of patients anticipating their examinations. In this example, such a backup has occurred, and by the time the patient begins her procedure, she is almost hysterical and has difficulty following the mammographer's directions. Her inability to hold still and endure the compression necessitates retakes of the films. By the time the woman is finished with the examination, she is angry and vows never to return to the breast imaging center. Her anger may even prevent her from following through with future mammograms.

Discussion questions

- What problems have occurred in this scenario?
- Whose problems are they, and what are the possible solutions?
- What impact has caring or the lack of it had on the ethical dilemma facing the mammographer?

Imaging professionals are not capable of providing perfect care. However, in striving for the ideal, the imaging professional may occasionally come close to achieving it and in so doing provide great benefits for the patient. Nevertheless, one danger in discussing ideals is viewing them as achievable and measurable commodities; this leads to the idea that those who fall short of achieving ideal care should be ashamed.[7] This misperception may lead imaging professionals who consider caring to be a vital part of their professional practice to feel guilty, selfish, or discouraged when they are unable to give more time to their patients.[9]

Obstacles to Caring

Imaging professionals face a variety of obstacles to providing caring treatment:

- Scarcity of time
- Technical priorities
- Impact of personal life
- Lack of training in caring for patients who are critically or terminally ill
- Lack of communication
- Societal pressures
- Lack of faith in self

All these obstacles lend themselves to personal and professional ethical dilemmas. Imaging professionals who feel inadequate as a result of any of these obstacles may have difficulty feeling or expressing caring.

PROFESSIONAL CARE

Professional care is characterized by the application of the knowledge of a professional discipline, including its science, theory, practice, and art. It is complementary to human caring. Imaging professionals must possess human caring before they are able to provide professional caring. Human and professional caring are both activities of the whole person (although activities are only a portion of caring). The interaction of compassion, knowledge, and the experiences and emotions of the whole person give rise to human and professional caring.[7]

PROFESSIONAL CARE
Professional care is the application of the knowledge of a discipline, including its science, theory, practice, and art.

Clearly, professional expertise unaccompanied by human compassion is not enough to serve all the needs of the patient: "If we fail to motivate that feeling (empathy and compassion) and the earnest desire within our student to help our fellow man, we will have created the equivalent of human robots."[10] Such an emphasis on skill at the expense of caring and empathy produces a "patient-care gap" in which the patient is ignored as the "scale tips toward science and technique."[11]

Caring in the Imaging Sciences

The professional and human caring practiced by imaging professionals is based on individual and institutional values. Adherence to a set of values and the use of ethical problem solving aid the imaging professional in developing a more caring demeanor. The three strengthen one another: without values, caring and ethics in the imaging health care environment are without foundation and force. In turn, a strong commitment to caring requires a fusing of feeling, thought, and action, all of which aid the technologist in coping with stress and solving problems ethically.

Taken together, caring, values, and ethical problem solving give meaning to professional practice, create the possibility of ever-improving care, and enhance patient comfort and feelings of safety.[2] For example, cardiac ultrasonographers who have the ability to make their patients comfortable find them more willing to comply with directions, thus allowing a more diagnostic examination.

Caring brings together all the resources of the imaging professional. When imaging professionals care for patients by performing imaging procedures, monitoring equipment, and providing for patient needs, they do more than provide therapy; they become a part of the patient's life.

Caring in the imaging sciences also involves an appreciation of the universal patterns of human experience. As imaging students enter educational programs, they are exposed through their patients to the universality of pain, loneliness, suffering, fear, and looming death. Human and professional caring require compassion for the suffering endured by patients and an understanding of the ways in which people construct their lives and draw meaning from them. This unending activity of inventing, restructuring, and reinterpreting is universal, even though the outcomes are personal. Compassionate imaging professionals respond to the universal appeal made by suffering human beings by caring, the potential for which is universal as well.[7]

Imaging professionals see patients in all phases of life and all conditions of health and disease. Because the nature of their practice requires care for a diverse patient population, imaging educational programs incorporate classes in caring skill development. However, professionals in other modalities who may not have as much continued and direct contact with a wide variety of patients may not be as prepared to care. This disparity may be an obstacle to providing the safe, comfortable environment patients require.

Careful monitoring of radiologic equipment is another activity that shows caring by ensuring the autonomy, comfort, and safety of the patient. Quality control specialists exhibit caring by spending as much time as necessary monitoring imaging machinery. Imaging professionals also show caring for their patients by ensuring confidentiality, obtaining informed consent, thoroughly explaining procedures, and taking complete and accurate histories. Human and professional caring are exhibited by nuclear medicine technologists who explain the significance of the radioactive material being injected into a patient receiving a therapeutic dose.

Developing a More Caring Demeanor

Caring is an attitude that may be developed and learned (Figure 9-1). Courses in professional caring have been part of the radiologic sciences curriculum for some time. However, education in human caring and human relations skills development are somewhat newer additions to the curriculum. To enhance caring, imaging professionals must strengthen and integrate their mental, physical, and spiritual capacities. By learning all they can about professional practice and human interaction, loving more, and being more creative and generous in spirit, imaging professionals can improve their ability to evaluate and solve ethical and technical problems. Self-analysis and rating of caring abilities provide further insights into caring strengths and weaknesses.

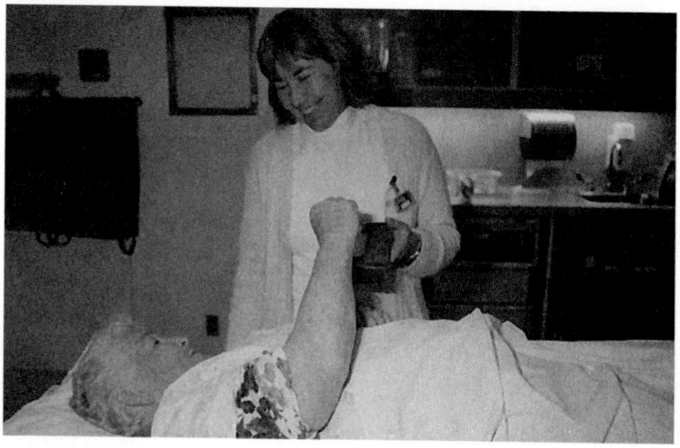

FIGURE 9-1
A caring demeanor can be expressed through helping, nurturing, and offering support.

Imaging programs can use a variety of means to instill a desire to increase caring skills in students:

- Communications classes that address body language and the importance of listening
- Critical thinking classes that focus on recognizing, analyzing, and evaluating ethical dilemmas
- Discussions of films that illustrate caring scenarios (e.g., *The Doctor*)
- Empathy rotations that require students to become patients for a day and participate in a variety of imaging patient activities
- Role-modeling by instructors and staff technologists, including student evaluation
- Discussions among classmates of hospitalization and health care provider experiences, with an emphasis on the ways in which caring influences outcomes
- A review of patient interviews in which care needs are identified and the department's response to those needs is evaluated
- Review and discussion of educational and professional materials dealing with issues of caring

EXAMPLES OF CARING

Each of the following examples provides an illustration of caring. They demonstrate the ways in which this essential human quality is finely honed by professional training and expressed humanly rather than perfectly. They depict imaging professionals engaged with the whole of their professional knowledge, as well as their human spirits.

Neurointensive Care Unit

Jane Smith is a radiographer in charge of portable imaging, and one of her patients is a young man who is an illegal immigrant. He has been in a car accident and has a serious head injury. He has no family in this country. The patient has been unconscious since his accident. Smith is quite concerned about the well-being of this patient, and though she does not condone his illegal status, she does not feel it is relevant to the situation. She realizes that she must monitor every change in the patient's condition when she is taking his radiographs. She watches all the radiographic equipment carefully. She also uses all her physical assessment skills to detect any complications that may arise. She talks to him in an attempt to stimulate his mind and penetrate his coma while performing his radiographs. He cannot talk to her, however, and may not even be aware of her care. Nonetheless, the imaging professional feels it is her duty to use her whole person on behalf of the patient's well-being—to care.[12]

Oncology Unit

Mike Jones, a radiation therapist, is the primary therapist for a 53-year-old grandmother who has advanced cancer. She is in pain and aware that her prognosis is poor. While Jones is positioning her, she says to him, "Are you a religious man, Mike?" Actually, Jones does not consider himself a particularly religious man, and furthermore he has much to do this morning. He is inwardly annoyed at being called on to enter into this patient's suffering; this morning, at least, he would rather attend to other things. He is a human being and not capable of providing perfect care. However, he recognizes that religion is not the issue here; rather, the patient is seeking a human connection and comfort in her fear.

He sits down beside her to signal his intention to be fully present to her and enter into her experience, not because he plans to stay a long time. Human interaction need not always take a long time. Speaking truthfully, he says, "My own religion has its ups and downs—does yours provide you some comfort now?" The question is gentle and undemanding. The patient may choose to speak briefly about her religion and remain silent about other concerns. However, she also may choose to accept and respond to his gentle acknowledgment of her need for comfort. She replies, "I know that I have not much longer to live. I long to watch my grandchild grow up a bit longer and offer more support to his parents. My comfort is in knowing that the Lord does things in His own good time and that He will provide for my children." Jones takes her hand for a moment and says, "Your faith that the Lord will provide for your children seems a comfort to you now indeed." His answer is brief and tacitly accepting of everything she has said. He waits to see if she needs any further support, and she pats his hand and says, "Well, you have others to take care of. Thank you so much."[12]

LEGAL ISSUES

LEGAL SIDE OF CARING

Caring may not appear to be a topic with many legal implications, and strictly speaking this is true. However, a review of the many legal issues previously discussed reveals that patient care does indeed have legal aspects. No federal or state statutes define or mandate caring; no complainant will ever attempt to make a prima facie case of "not caring." Because of this lack of legal guidance, imaging professionals must use a common-sense approach when caring for patients. Indeed, patients are more likely to file a malpractice suit when they are unhappy with the "care" they received, so there is a practical aspect to caring.

For example, researchers from Harvard University reviewed more than 31,000 New York hospital records from 1984 to determine the incidence of injuries resulting from medical negligence.[13] This study found that the incidence of adverse events caused by negligence during hospitalizations in New York in 1984 was 3.7%. In studying the litigation data for the same year, the researchers also found that eight times as many patients suffered an injury from negligence as filed a malpractice suit, and that about sixteen times as many patients suffered an injury from negligence as received compensation.

These data indicate that most patients injured as a result of negligence do not file malpractice claims. Patient dissatisfaction has been linked with the filing of medical malpractice claims. Generally, patients do not consult an attorney unless they are unhappy with the "care" they receive.

Caring, then, may be the single most important thing the imaging professional can do to minimize the risk of litigation. Imaging professionals can do their best to ensure their patients understand the procedures and are able to give truly informed consent. Imaging professionals also can do their best to follow procedures with the goal of obtaining maximal studies, providing minimal radiation exposure, and keeping patients safe.

However, imaging professionals, physicians, and patients are all human, and no human being is perfect. Mistakes sometimes happen, and things sometimes do not go as they should. Generally, it is patients who are dissatisfied with the "caring" they received who seek legal recourse when these mistakes happen.

Probably the most important benefit gained in caring for patients is the patient's knowledge of the professional's care. As stated earlier in this chapter, imaging professionals must be part scientist, part humanist. Imaging professionals who share their humanist sides with patients by caring go a long way toward minimizing the risks of litigation.

SUMMARY

Caring is crucial in the development of the imaging professional. It is essential to the treatment provided in the imaging environment and the ethical problem solving required to provide quality imaging services.

Caring is a function of the whole person in which concern for the growth and well-being of another is expressed in an integrated application of the mind, body, and spirit that seeks to maximize positive outcomes. Existential care is compassion arising from an awareness of common bonds of humanity and common expressions, fates, and feelings. Professional care is the application of the knowledge of the discipline, including its science, theory, practice, and art. Human and professional caring in the imaging sciences provide safety and comfort for patients, involve imaging professionals in their patients' lives, and enhance patient autonomy, confidentiality, and informed consent.

Education to enhance caring may be incorporated into the imaging curriculum in a variety of methods. By developing more caring demeanors, imaging professionals become better able to provide patients with compassionate treatment and quality imaging services. Caring is therefore an ethical imperative in the radiologic sciences.

Litigation risks are also decreased by imaging professionals who care. Patient dissatisfaction is linked to the filing of medical malpractice claims. Generally, patients do not consult an attorney unless they are unhappy with the "care" they received.

ENDNOTES

1. Erickson E: *The life cycle completed,* New York, 1982, W.W. Norton.
2. Griffin AP: A philosophical analysis of caring in nursing, *J Adv Nurs* 8:289, 1983.
3. Warren L: Review and synthesis of nine nursing studies on care and caring, *J NY State Nurs Assoc* 19(4):17, 1988.
4. Gaut D: Development of a theoretically adequate description of caring, *West J Nurs Res* 5(4):311, 1983.
5. Leininger M: The phenomenon of caring: importance, research questions and theoretical considerations. In Leininger M, editor: *Caring: an essential human need,* Thorofare, NJ, 1988, Slack.
6. Dowd S: The radiographer's role: part scientist, part humanist, *Radiol Technol* 63(4):240, 1992.
7. Younger J: Literary works as a mode of knowledge, *Image: J Nurs Scholar* 22(1):39, 1990.
8. Stumpfig K: Caring can't be scheduled, *Radiol Technol* 66(3):208, 1995.
9. Dowd S: Do we care?, *RT Image* 3:16, 1990.
10. Ohnysty J: *Aids to ethics and professional conduct for student radiographers,* Springfield, Ill., 1968, Charles C. Thomas.
11. Fengler K: The patient care gap, *Radiol Technol* 49:599, 1978.
12. Creasia JL, Parker B: *Conceptual foundations of professional nursing practice,* ed 2, St Louis, 1996, Mosby.
13. Furrow B et al: *Liability and quality issues in health care,* St. Paul, Minn., 1991, West.

REVIEW QUESTIONS

1 Define *human caring.*
2 Define *professional care.*
3 Define *existential care.*
4 Imaging professionals must provide __________ __________ in addition to professional caring to satisfy the needs of the patient.
5 Caring is an __________ analogous to truth and justice.
6 List some of the obstacles to caring.
7 The human caring practiced by professionals is based on _____ and _____ values.
8 List three methods of developing caring skills.
9 Explain the ways in which advocacy influences care for the imaging patient.
10 **True or False** Caring involves initiative.
11 **True or False** A more caring demeanor cannot be developed.
12 **True or False** An ethical approach to problem solving is an expression of caring.
13 **True or False** Time constraints may have a detrimental effect on patient satisfaction.
14 **True or False** Caring can be fully attained with perfect human expression.
15 **True or False** The lack of training in caring for critically ill patients is an obstacle to caring.
16 **True or False** Most patients do not consult an attorney unless they are unhappy with the "care" they received.
17 **True or False** Because of the lack of legal guidance, imaging professionals must use a common-sense approach when caring for patients.
18 **True or False** "Caring" has no relationship to minimizing the risk of litigation.
19 **True or False** Federal and state statutes define and mandate caring.
20 **True or False** Most patients injured as a result of negligence file malpractice suits.
21 **True or False** Patient dissatisfaction has been linked with the filing of malpractice claims.

CRITICAL THINKING QUESTIONS & ACTIVITIES

1 Is involvement in the universal conditions of life experienced by patients an important aspect of caring? Defend your answer.

2 The technical aspects of providing imaging services for patients may adversely affect the human caring delivered by the imaging professional. Give an example of this and justify your reasoning.

3 In what way does the appropriate taking of a patient's history enhance caring? Why?

4 List the resources of the imaging professional that enable caring for the patient. In what way do they enable caring?

5 Why is caring the foundation of the imaging services?

PROFESSIONAL PROFILE

A SONOGRAPHER WAS CALLED in to perform a pelvic sonogram to rule out ectopic pregnancy. The examination was performed and sent for interpretation via teleradiology. The radiologist discussed the case with the sonographer and stated that it was an intrauterine pregnancy and told the sonographer to contact the emergency room (ER) and convey the findings. The sonographer called the ER, told the unit clerk it was an intrauterine pregnancy, and then went home.

The next day the sonographer was called into the supervisor's office and informed that the unit clerk had told the ER physician that the patient had an ectopic pregnancy. The sonographer explained that she had told the unit clerk it was a normal pregnancy.

Always provide a written report of findings for call-back procedures. For teleradiology, the sonographer should write down the physician's findings, read them back, and list the physician's name, time of report, and the name of the sonographer who transcribed the report. If an oral report is also given, list the name of the person taking the report and include the content of the report that was given. This will minimize the likelihood of false reports and prevent the situation of one person's word against another's, always a tenuous situation.

BETH ANDERHUB, MEd, RDMS
DIRECTOR, ULTRASOUND PROGRAM
ST. LOUIS COMMUNITY COLLEGE
St. Louis, Missouri

CHAPTER 10

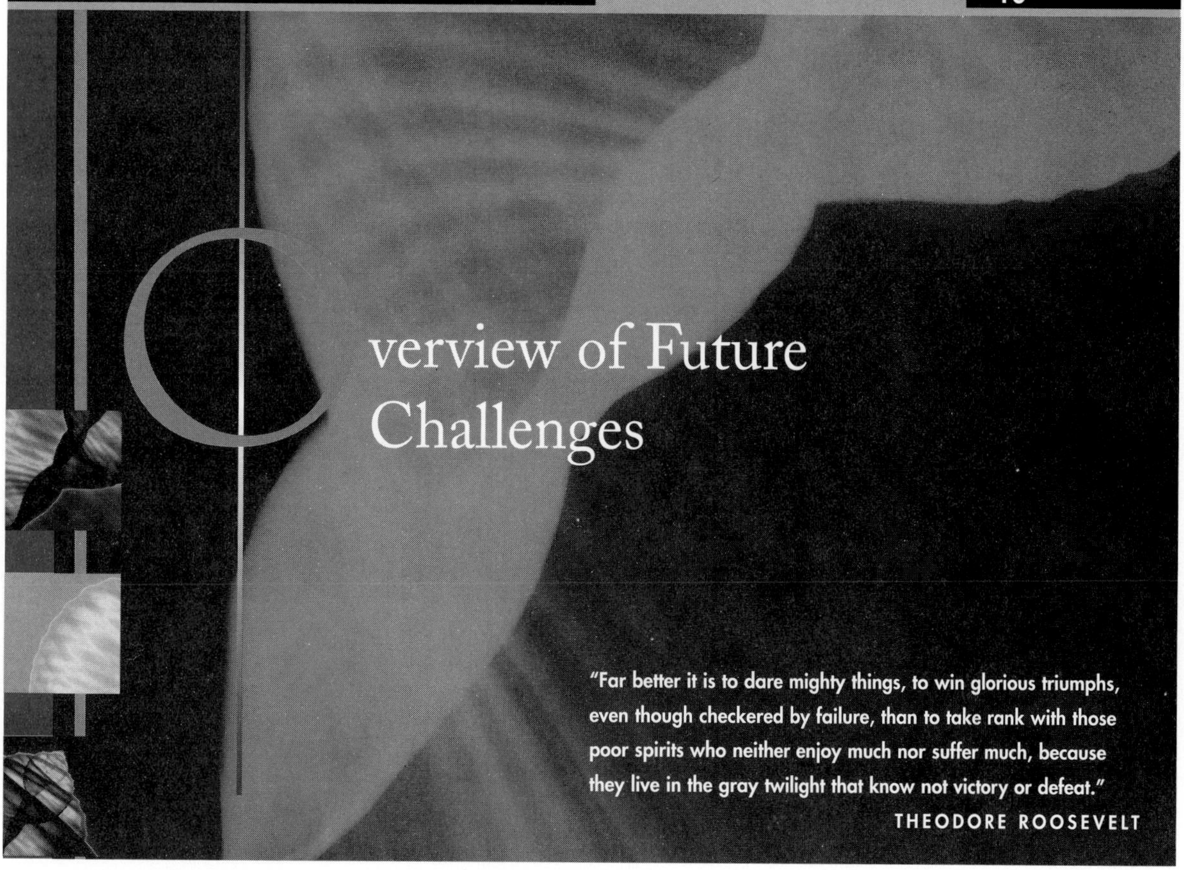

Overview of Future Challenges

"Far better it is to dare mighty things, to win glorious triumphs, even though checkered by failure, than to take rank with those poor spirits who neither enjoy much nor suffer much, because they live in the gray twilight that know not victory or defeat."

THEODORE ROOSEVELT

LEARNING OBJECTIVES

- Recognize the variety of ethical challenges for imaging professionals arising from the following areas:
  - Research methodology
  - Radiographic interpretation and testing
  - Transplant situations
  - New reproductive methods
  - Quality control and improvement
- Recognize and identify the complex legal and ethical issues raised by changing technologies.
- Discuss the inability of law to act proactively in changing technologic fields.
- Understand the guidelines provided by professional organizations to aid in ethical decision making in controversial situations.

CHAPTER OUTLINE

ETHICAL ISSUES

The previous chapters of this text have discussed ethical concepts, theories, and common problems faced by radiographers. However, the problems discussed are not the only ethical dilemmas encountered by radiographers. Moreover, as the imaging profession and medical technology evolve, imaging professionals will face intense new ethical problems requiring strong problem-solving skills. Considerations of research methodology, new reproductive methods, testing, transplant situations, and quality control and improvement require professionals to have ethical awareness of their possible abuses and controversies to provide the best possible patient care.

Imaging professionals should be prepared to encounter a variety of new difficulties on the path to ethical problem solving. This chapter offers a brief overview of ethical areas in which radiographers may become involved.

BIOMEDICAL RESEARCH

Imaging professionals may be employed by institutions that conduct research on human beings. Certain imaging examinations such as chest radiographs, high-speed radiographs, and nuclear scans may be performed on experimental subjects to ascertain the effect of experimental drugs or treatments. Ethical dilemmas may arise if imaging specialists are concerned about the ways in which subjects are influenced to consent to the research study. Imaging specialists also may wonder whether the risks taken by experimental subjects are justified by the possible benefits to society.

Research may be expensive. The expense involved should produce good proportionate to the evils risked to be considered ethical and justified.

THE IMAGING PROFESSIONAL'S OBLIGATION TO RESEARCH

Imaging professionals have an obligation to the profession to maintain current knowledge and be critically aware of future technology and trends. This maintenance and education requires imaging professionals to read scientific journals and practice proper research methods. While reviewing various research materials, imaging professionals must analyze the data and practice critical thinking (see Box 1-1).

Imaging professionals concerned with respect and stature in the health care community should consider the options available to them to encourage others to perceive them more positively. They should educate others about the profession and describe the creative and innovative processes they have undertaken and completed. Moreover, they should expend the extra effort to describe their findings and experiences in established journals. Imaging educators should encourage and require their students to perform and present research; unfortunately, the imaging sciences lag behind medicine and nursing in research and publishing. Professional journals, periodicals, and organizations are eager for imaging professionals and students to submit work. Given this desire for information and education, imaging professionals must look to the future and encourage the recognition of the imaging sciences.[1]

ETHICS OF INTERPRETATION OF IMAGING PROCEDURES AND TESTING

Imaging procedures in all modalities require interpretation. Many imaging professionals have observed differences of opinion between radiologists and physicians concerning the characteristics of a quality image. An internist may see a fracture and begin treatment for it. A radiologist may look at the same image and read it as negative. Such fallibility of interpretation may cause technologists to become involved in litigation.

Other imaging professionals may be asked by physicians or emergency personnel to make judgment calls concerning the outcome of tests or imaging procedures. Although the imaging technologist may feel an image clearly shows a fractured bone, basing treatment for a fracture on the opinion of a professional who is not a radiologist may not be fair to the patient.

A less common dilemma encountered by imaging professionals occurs when they know or at least perceive that a test has been misinterpreted. Such a situation raises the question of the responsibilities a technologist has to a patient who has an undiagnosed

IMAGING SCENARIO

A radiographer who had been hired only recently was called to the morgue to take a series of skull radiographs on a body for forensic evaluation. The county medical examiner was present and remarked that no evidence on the films indicated foul play. The radiographer, however, noted an unnatural line on the basal skull projection. The new employee was afraid to say anything to the medical examiner and thus waited until the next day to talk to the radiologist. The radiologist read the examination as positive for fracture, but he was not inclined to call the medical examiner because of a previous confrontation with the examiner. However, he did ask the radiographer why he had not pointed out the suspicious line to the examiner. The radiographer explained that he did not believe he was qualified to interpret films. After the medical examiner received the radiologist's report, he was furious because he had already released the body and it had been cremated. He cornered the radiographer later that same day and asked him directly if he had noticed the fracture line. The radiographer admitted with a great deal of hesitation that he had seen the fracture. The medical examiner accused the radiographer of negligence and explained that if the person had been killed that the murderer would go unpunished. The family of the deceased, after being informed by an anonymous source, later sued the medical examiner, radiologist, and radiographer.

Discussion questions

- Who was to blame?
- What alternatives did the individuals involved have?
- Should all three health care providers have been sued?
- What ethical theory would provide the best tool for answering these ethical questions? Why?
- What would you have done? (Remember, this person was a new employee.)

fracture and is being sent home from the emergency room. The risks to the patient outweigh the risks to the imaging professional, indicating that the professional should intervene. This intervention may require little more than questioning a line on the cervical body. Imaging professionals who intervene on behalf of patients in what they believe is the patients' best interests may put themselves at risk. However, if the benefits outweigh the risks, imaging professionals may choose to intervene.

Imaging testing includes nonmedical testing and industrial testing as well. These noninvasive tests involve evaluating pipe lines, casting, and fittings for their strength and structure. Other types of radiographic testing include forensic radiography on human subjects or objects to solve crimes. Archaeological imaging has aided in examining mummified remains and exploring remains of previous civilizations. Imaging studies of art objects also have proved invaluable in discovering forgeries. Truthfulness and disclosure are as important in these nonmedical imaging areas as they are in medical imaging practice.

ETHICAL DILEMMAS OF TRANSPLANTS

Imaging professionals may find themselves involved with patients and families awaiting organ transplants; they also may have contact with donors and their families. The events surrounding organ transplantation often are emotional and must be handled with empathy and ethical awareness (Box 10-1).

IMAGING SCENARIO

An imaging professional employed by a major oil company was responsible for producing radiographic images of the newly placed pipeline. As the professional surveyed the results of his latest work, he noticed a crack in the pipeline along with several other imaging artifacts. He approached his supervisor with the information. The supervisor, who was being pressured by the company's owners to expedite the process because of issues of time and money, questioned the results of the study.

The questionable findings were pigeonholed on the supervisor's desk. The imaging professional decided to go to the company's owners and share his concerns. Before he could keep this appointment, he was terminated because of the quality of his work and denied references.

Discussion questions

- What would the next step be for the industrial technologist?
- What values are in conflict?
- In what way do ethical and legal issues influence this situation?

BOX 10-1 CONSIDERATIONS IN TRANSPLANT ETHICS

1. Obtaining of appropriate informed consent
2. Respectful empathy for the emotional precariousness of patients and families
3. Provision of quality care to donor and recipient

The AMA Council on Ethical and Judicial Affairs has outlined the principal ethical concerns of the physician and health care team—including the radiographer[2]:

1. Full discussion of the proposed procedure with the donor and recipient or responsible relatives or representatives is mandatory. The physician should be objective in discussing the procedure, disclosing known risks and possible hazards, and advising of the alternative procedures available. The physician should not encourage expectations beyond those justified by the circumstances. The physician's interest in advancing scientific knowledge must always be secondary to the primary concern for the patient.
2. The transplantation of body organs should be undertaken only by physicians who possess special medical knowledge and technical competence developed through special training, study, and laboratory experience and practice. Transplants must take place in medical institutions with facilities adequate to protect the health and well-being of the parties to the procedure.
3. Transplantation of body organs should be undertaken only after careful evaluation of the availability and effectiveness of other possible therapy.

Ethical concerns raised by transplant situations involve the obtaining of informed consent, the avoidance of playing on the emotions of the families and patients involved, the proposing of any viable alternatives, the provision of appropriate care to brain-dead donors even if a transplant is anticipated, and above all the maintenance of basic protections for donors and patients[1]:

> In the face of the shortage of organs and the urgency of many situations, there are proposals to increase the supply of organs by improving the recruitment of volunteers and by changing the legal requirements for surrogate consent. The methods proposed pose their own ethical problems.

Nuclear medicine personnel may certainly find themselves involved in transplant situations. Nuclear medicine involves the injection of radioactive materials into the body. Pathology may be discovered through the observance of images of the radioactive material's uptake, use, and excretion by the body. Nuclear medicine technologists often are involved in obtaining images of brain function and may be involved in considerations of brain death because nuclear medicine brain imaging may be used to help determine brain death.

IMAGING SCENARIO

A young man suffering massive head trauma from a motorcycle accident is brought to the emergency room. He is unresponsive and has a flat electroencephalogram. A nuclear study is ordered as a necessary criterion to determine brain death.

In the same hospital, a young woman lies in dire need of a liver. She may die within the next few days if she does not receive a transplant. The family of the young man wants to do everything possible to keep the patient alive,

IMAGING SCENARIO—cont'd

but the nuclear study reveals no brain function. The family is approached by various hospital personnel to consider donating the young man's organs. However, the family is unwilling to suspend life support and donate the organs. The nuclear technologist feels comfortable enough with the young man's family to discuss organ donation with them. When family members question the technologist, she is tempted to use every method possible to convince them that their son will not recover and they should donate his organs.

Discussion questions

- Whose purpose is the nuclear technologist serving—that of the patient, the woman needing a liver, or her own conscience?
- What are ethical implications of harvesting the organs from a body still functioning on life support?
- When does death occur?
- When has all hope been exhausted?
- Whose hope is more important—that of the family of the potential donor or that of the potential recipient?

NEW REPRODUCTIVE METHODS

Ultrasonographers tend to be more involved with the ethical dilemmas presented by new reproductive methods than other imaging specialists. Infertility treatments have progressed tremendously over the past several years, and ultrasonographers currently play an important role in such procedures. Ultrasonography allows the visualization of the follicles. Doppler studies indicate blood flow to the ovum. Other imaging professionals take part in certain procedures used for diagnosing infertility such as hysterosalpingography and urethrograms.

A number of ethical dilemmas arise from new reproductive methods (Box 10-2). Each of these dilemmas must be studied in depth and addressed on its own merits; this overview does not undertake this task. Imaging professionals involved in these controversies would benefit from a personal study of reproductive method ethics.

Imaging professionals should participate in medically indicated diagnostic procedures as long as the appropriate informed consent procedures have been employed. However, they should be wary of the possible abuses of new technologies, and they have a right to refuse to take part in frivolous or cavalier procedures.

Imaging professionals also have a right not to participate in procedures they do not condone such as abortions. However, if imaging professionals are aware that part of their employment practice involves providing this type of care, they need to determine whether they should provide this service or seek employment elsewhere. In addition, they should not place themselves in the position of deciding whether a patient should have such a procedure.

BOX 10-2 ETHICAL DILEMMAS IN ASSISTED REPRODUCTION

Artificial insemination
Surrogate mothers
Risks to mother and child
Donor concealment and the right to privacy
In vitro fertilization
Embryo transfers
Charges of artificiality
Use of frozen embryos and sperm banks
Reimbursement for surrogacy and donation of eggs and sperm

CONTINUOUS QUALITY IMPROVEMENT AND QUALITY CONTROL

CONTINUOUS QUALITY IMPROVEMENT
The aspect of quality assurance that monitors technical equipment to maintain quality standards.

Quality control and *continuous quality improvement* are health care buzzwords of the 1990s. The growing emphasis on the maintenance and improvement of quality of care has influenced the ethics of problem solving. The incorporation of problem-solving methods into quality control programs has produced the management philosophy of total quality improvement. Quality improvement programs seek to anticipate problems by data gathering and trend analysis and improve the environment before problems arise.

The need for quality improvement programs is clear[3]:

> A test result lost, a specialist who cannot be reached, a missing requisition, a misinterpreted order, duplicate paperwork, a vanished record, a long wait for the [computed tomography] CT scan, an unreliable on-call system—these are all-too-familiar examples of waste, rework, complexity, and error in the doctor's daily life. . . . For the average doctor, quality fails when systems fail.

The same holds true for all health care providers, including imaging professionals. Quality assurance and quality improvement programs focus on the best interests of patients. Imaging professionals can aid in this patient-focused striving for quality care by enhancing their ethical awareness and problem-solving skills. The combination of quality improvement programs with professional ethics allows imaging departments to serve both patient and organizational needs. For more information and practical methods, Dr. Jeffrey Papp's *Quality Management in the Imaging Technologies* offers an in-depth examination of continuous quality as it applies to all modalities in the imaging sciences.[4]

ETHICS COMMITTEES

Many institutions have an ethics committee composed of physicians, chaplains, administrative personnel, and employees from various departments. Legal representatives may also be involved. These committees serve as problem-solving and decision-making bodies. When an ethical dilemma arises that cannot be resolved at a personal or departmental level, the committee chooses a course of action based

IMAGING SCENARIO

A sonographer has been working with a couple for the treatment of infertility. In the course of their relationship over the preceding 10 months, they have become close. Unfortunately, after 10 months of treatment, the couple's chances of pregnancy appear slim.

In the eleventh month of treatment, fertilization is successful and an embryo is formed. The couple and sonographer are overjoyed. The waiting and hoping are over. The thousands of dollars—almost their entire savings—have paid off. If anyone deserves this miracle, they do. They have had an exceptionally difficult time with the procedures and have been emotionally spent for nearly a year.

However, genetic testing of the embryo reveals a problem. A few missing chromosomes have left a pattern that indicates the child may be born with Williams syndrome. This condition produces mild-to-severe mental retardation; genetic testing cannot predict the level of impairment. Williams syndrome also entails health problems such as heart abnormalities and organ dysfunctions.

The physician discusses the situation with the couple, and they are devastated. He encourages them to abort and try again.

When the couple arrive for a sonographic examination to determine fetal age, they share the unhappy news with the sonographer, who is dismayed by their consideration of abortion. He has a younger brother with Williams syndrome and loves him very much. His interactions with his brother have made him aware both of the difficulties and joys of having a special brother. When the couple ask him for his opinion, he must decide whether to share his personal experiences with them.

Discussion questions

- How much of his personal life should he share?
- Will the couple's care be compromised if the sonographer's remarks contradict those of the physician?
- Can the couple emotionally and financially afford the abortive procedure and another attempt to produce an embryo?
- Should they take their chances with the fetus they have?
- Should they consider adoption?
- How would you deal with this situation if you were the sonographer?

on its best collaborative judgment of what ought to be done. This decision is based on institutional values, personal values, and the moral meaning of the situation to all parties involved.

Imaging professionals may become involved in ethics committees, especially when ethical dilemmas present themselves in the imaging environment (Box 10-3).

BOX 10-3 ETHICS COMMITTEES FOR THE FUTURE

The year is 2026, and the imaging center is bustling with activity. As the imaging supervisor reviews the day's procedures and determines the units to activate, the patients are aligned for entrance into the imaging dome. The dome was recently leased from the sole provider of imaging equipment. After managed care led to monopolies for technology providers and the federal government intervened to regulate health care costs, the purchasing of equipment became much less time consuming and often less expensive.

Robotic units gently transport the patients as their audio programs explain the procedures, obtain informed consent, and install the patients in the imaging dome, a small room containing all the necessary scanning and recording equipment. As patients enter the room, their vital signs are recorded; within 60 seconds the machinery performs a total-body scan, including lab scanning. The scanned images are then relayed to the master reader at the state capital, and the images and reports are sent to the physicians' and patients' personal modems within a few seconds.

All imaging is noninvasive and nonionizing. Thermal, ultrasound, and magnetic imaging are used simultaneously as patients revolve on a platform in the imaging dome and projections are made at every conceivable angle. All procedures involve total-body imaging so that all patient information is provided and patients do not have the ability to conceal any health information the federal imaging center might find useful to determine the patient's treatment needs.

The first group of patients for the day are cloned specimens to be evaluated for transplant fitness. The second group are geriatric patients. Because the prescribed life expectancy is 120 years, geriatric patients are evaluated for the euthanasia program. The next group of patients are pregnant women whose fetuses are to be studied to determine viability. Fetuses determined to be unfit for mental or physical reasons are aborted and used for organ transplants. Patients with traumatic injuries are evaluated with portable domes and triaged to determine cost benefits.

As the imaging supervisor completes the last of the day's procedures, she remembers that she has an ethical and legal issues committee meeting at the capital center.

Discussion questions

- What sort of issues would be discussed at such a meeting?
- In what ways have the ethical and legal issues changed since the twentieth century?
- Why have these changes occurred?
- In what ways do ethics and law change with technology?

LEGAL ISSUES

Technology is changing at such a rapid rate that the scenario described in Box 10-3 may not be all that implausible. With this changing technology, new and more complex legal issues arise. Legislatures attempt to write statutes that consider at least foreseeable technologic changes. Judicial decisions, however, are always based on a set of facts that has *already* occurred, and the ability to use judicial decisions in evaluating new technologies and the influence they have on human life is difficult. If clear legal opinions are not available, policies developed by professional medical organizations are often used as guidelines.

The effect of new technologies on imaging professionals will be varied and is currently largely unknown. Imaging professionals are and will continue to be involved in new developments in technology, although the nature of that involvement is difficult to predict. The possibilities are endless, including ultrasonography connected with more advanced assisted conception; imaging and evaluation of clone organs for possible transplantation; and ultrasonography used for selective abortion based on genetic testing. Guidance must be sought from the scientific community and professional organizations to ensure that these advances will be used for the good of all.

THE LAW AND THE FUTURE

Where does the law of the future originate? With technology advancing rapidly, legislatures cannot foresee the consequences of that technology and make appropriate statutory changes to deal with them. Judicial decisions, because they are based on past sets of facts, are of little assistance in dealing with a technologically advanced future. Where then, do the courts look for guidance?

Many professional organizations exist within the medical community. Members of these organizations spend countless hours grappling with ethical and legal consequences of the technological advances of their particular specialties. Legislatures turn to these organizations for guidance in drafting legislation, and courts often turn to them for guidance when attempting to sort out issues that never before existed.

One such example of the guidance available to legislators is the Uniform Status of Children of Assisted Conception Act (The Act).[5] The Act was drafted as a model for states to use in drafting their own statutes to deal with this new technology. The following situation is cited as one of the primary reasons for the drafting of the Act.

It is now technologically possible to take the sperm from one source and the ovum from another, place the subsequently developed embryo in the uterus of a third person, and then have the child raised by two biologically unrelated persons. This raises the possibility of the child having five parents.[6] The purpose of the Act is to provide such a child with certainty as to his or her legal parentage.

Case Study

An example of the guidance used by the courts is the case of *Davis v Davis*.[7] This was the first case involving a pre-embryo (the product that results when an egg is fertilized by a sperm in a laboratory setting). In this case, the pre-embryos were frozen, the couple subsequently divorced, and a battle ensued over who, if anyone, should have custody of the frozen pre-embryos. The court looked to the guidance of the American Fertility Society and adopted their view that because of the potential of a pre-embryo to become a person, special respect is due.[7,8] The court thus recognized that the donors of the genetic material have an interest in the pre-embryos to the extent that they have decision-making authority concerning the disposition of the pre-embryos.

The guidance of the medical community is invaluable to legislators and courts. In the legal arena, where the usual statutes and precedents have little application, the knowledge and input of the medical community is the best source of information available. Professional organizations, most of which involve physicians and other health care workers who voluntarily give their time to these efforts, have the burden of monitoring technologic advances from an ethical standpoint to ensure that technology is used for good.

TECHNOLOGIC ADVANCES CAUSING LEGAL AND ETHICAL HAVOC

Assisted conception is one of the most advanced and fastest-changing areas of biomedicine; many imaging professionals are affected by this technology. However, advancements also are being made at amazing rates in other areas too numerous to cover here. Many of these new developments will also influence imaging professionals.

The implications to humankind of these technologies could be profound. Think about cloning, genetic testing that reveals everything about one's present and future physical condition, the ability to choose whether one's child will have green eyes or will be a superior athlete, and about the shortage and need for transplantable organs.

The legal and ethical issues are astounding. What legal rights would a human clone have? Is he or she able to give informed consent? Should we clone persons to supplement the supply of transplantable organs? Do employers and insurance companies have a right to the results of genetic testing that may show that we are prone to disease? Do human beings have the right to genetically engineer a child with certain physical attributes or talents? Do they have the right to dispose selectively of pre-embryos or abort embryos that do not have the desired characteristics?

The future, the unknown world of advancing technology, can be a frightening place. It is a place in which ethics and law need to interact to make some difficult choices. The law cannot be proactive to determine what is right for humankind in this world of advancing technology. Instead, imaging professionals must rely on ourselves as members of the scientific community and professional organizations to examine the ethical issues created by each advance and give our input to make those tough choices. The professional organizations that represent the imaging sciences are an important part of this scientific community.

ADVANCED TECHNOLOGY AND THE IMAGING PROFESSIONAL

The way these advances will affect the imaging professional is unclear. Imaging professionals will likely play an important role in many technologic advances. Examples include nuclear medicine technologists evaluating the organs of clones for possible transplantation and ultrasonographers assisting in abortions performed solely to select desired genetic traits.

Should it make a difference to the nuclear medicine technologist that the patient is a clone? Does a clone have a right to informed consent? Does it bother the ultrasonographer that he or she is assisting in the abortion of a fetus because it doesn't have the genes to excel in sports, be a rocket scientist, or have green eyes?

Future changes in technology will have a great impact on imaging professionals (Figure 10-1). They must look to the scientific community and its professional organizations to help form laws protecting the dignity of human life. Imaging professionals have responsibilities to remain aware of these advances. They must take an active role in the organizations representing the profession. These steps will allow them to remain aware and help their organizations take part in the examination of the technologies affecting the profession.

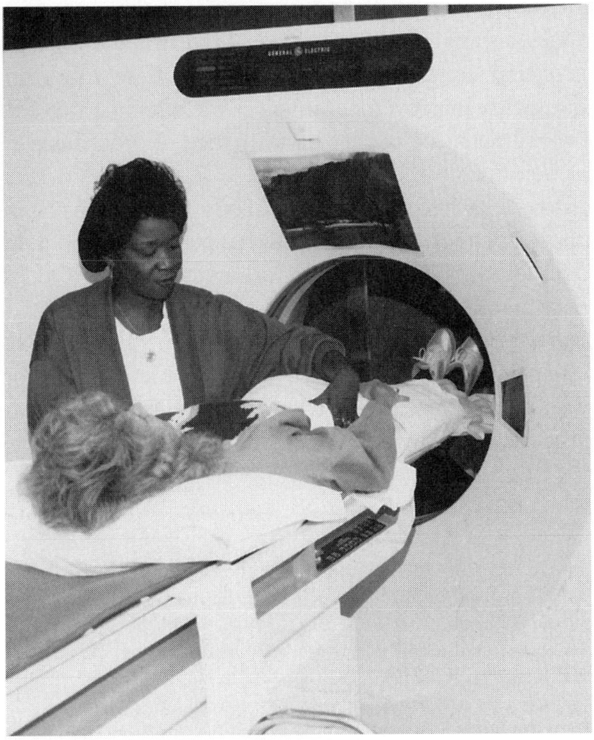

FIGURE 10-1
Keeping up with technologic advances is every imaging professional's responsibility.

SUMMARY

The rapid development of new technologies and the evolution of others presents imaging professionals with a variety of ethical dilemmas. These dilemmas may arise from research methodology, new reproductive methods, radiographic interpretation and testing, transplant situations, and quality control and quality improvement.

Research includes diagnostic radiography, high-speed radiography, nuclear medicine, and other modalities. Imaging professionals have an obligation to maintain current knowledge and be critically aware of future technology and trends.

New reproductive methods have created a host of ethical dilemmas. Ultrasonographers are confronted with these situations more often than other imaging professionals.

Interpretation of imaging procedures and tests often requires imaging professionals to employ ethical problem solving. Radiographers performing diagnostic radiography may become involved in situations involving physician misinterpretation of radiographic examinations. Imaging testing also may include industrial testing, forensic imaging, archaeological imaging, and imaging of art objects.

Organ transplant situations produce ethical dilemmas involving death and dying, informed consent, the offering of alternative treatments, the appropriate expression of empathy for families, and protection and adequate treatment for patients and donors.

Quality control and continuous quality improvement focus on the ethics of problem solving. Quality improvement involves the anticipation of the future needs of patients and consumers, the proper performance of procedures, and the correction of problems before they become serious.

Ethics committees may become involved in ethical problem solving. These committees are composed of a variety of institutional personnel who identify values and make the best decision possible for all parties involved.

The effect of technologic advances on imaging professionals is unclear. Future changes in technology will have a great impact on imaging professionals. Imaging professionals must continue to take an active role in the organizations representing the profession. This active participation allows imaging professionals to remain aware and help their organizations examine the technologies that will affect the profession.

ENDNOTES

1. Towsley-Cook D: An educator's voice—pride in the profession, *RT Image* 10(10):20, 1997.
2. AMA Council on Ethical and Judicial Affairs: *Current opinions of the Council on ethical and judicial affairs of the American Medical Association,* Chicago, 1986, AMA.
3. Joint Commission on Accreditation of Healthcare Organizations: *Transitions: from QA to CQI,* Oakbrook Terrace, Ill., 1991, JCAHO.
4. Papp J: *Quality management in the imaging sciences,* St Louis, 1998, Mosby.
5. Robinson R, Kurtz P: Uniform Status of Children of Assisted Conception Act: a view from the drafting committee, *Nova L Rev* 13:491, 1989.
6. Furrow B et al: *Health law,* St. Paul, Minn., 1995, West.
7. *Davis v Davis,* 842 S.W.2d 588 (Tenn. 1992).
8. American Fertility Society defines a pre-embryo as follows: "Pre-embryos are not persons, but because of their potential to become persons, they are entitled to special respect."

REVIEW QUESTIONS

1 The radiographer may become involved in ethical dilemmas concerned with which of the following?
   a. Biomedical research
   b. Reproduction methods
   c. Quality improvement
   d. All the above

2 Transplant situations require appropriate care for both the ________ ________ and ____________________ .

3 Why should imaging professionals be personally responsible for certain types of research? How does this display professionalism?

4 What are the attributes of a critical thinker? What skills do you need to develop to become a higher-level thinker?

5 Quality improvement addresses issues of ethics and patient care. Explain the ways in which the establishment of health care trends may improve patient care.

6 Why do imaging professionals need to anticipate and prepare for the ethical dilemmas of transplant procedures?

7 **True or False** Research methods involve critical thinking.

8 **True or False** Reading scientific journals is not a research method.

9 **True or False** The law is very clear on all reproductive issues.

10 **True or False** Laws are generally written for new technologies when those technologies are being developed.

11 **True or False** A good source of guidance in evolving technologic areas is the professional medical organization associated with that technology.

12 **True or False** The imaging professional has an obligation to stay abreast of technologic advances.

CRITICAL THINKING QUESTIONS & ACTIVITIES

1 Who should pay for the new methods of reproduction? Defend your answer.

2 How is the "good" of society helped or hindered by new methods of reproduction and imaging procedures and testing?

3 Analyze your own education and experience and the ways in which they prepared you for ethical awareness and decision making.

4 Examine your ethical strengths and weaknesses and the ways in which they aid and interfere with your ethical problem solving.

5 Interview an ethics committee member.

6 Establish an ethical awareness committee in your imaging area.

Continued

CRITICAL THINKING QUESTIONS & ACTIVITIES—cont'd

7 Describe imaging areas that are evolving and may face controversial ethical situations. Explain the situations.

8 Discuss a futuristic scenario in which you must perform an imaging procedure on a human clone to evaluate the donor liver before a liver transplant. Do you need to obtain informed consent? Is a clone a person?

9 Discuss a surrogacy situation in which the intended mother and father (whose ovum and sperm were used), the patient (the surrogate), and her husband all want to come in and view a sonographic examination of the surrogate. What should the sonographer do?

10 Discuss a scenario in which an ultrasonographer provides imaging services for a selective abortion because the parents want a child with the ability to become a concert pianist. Genetic testing has indicated that only the female of the three embryos has the concert pianist gene. Describe the ethical or legal problems with performing this procedure.

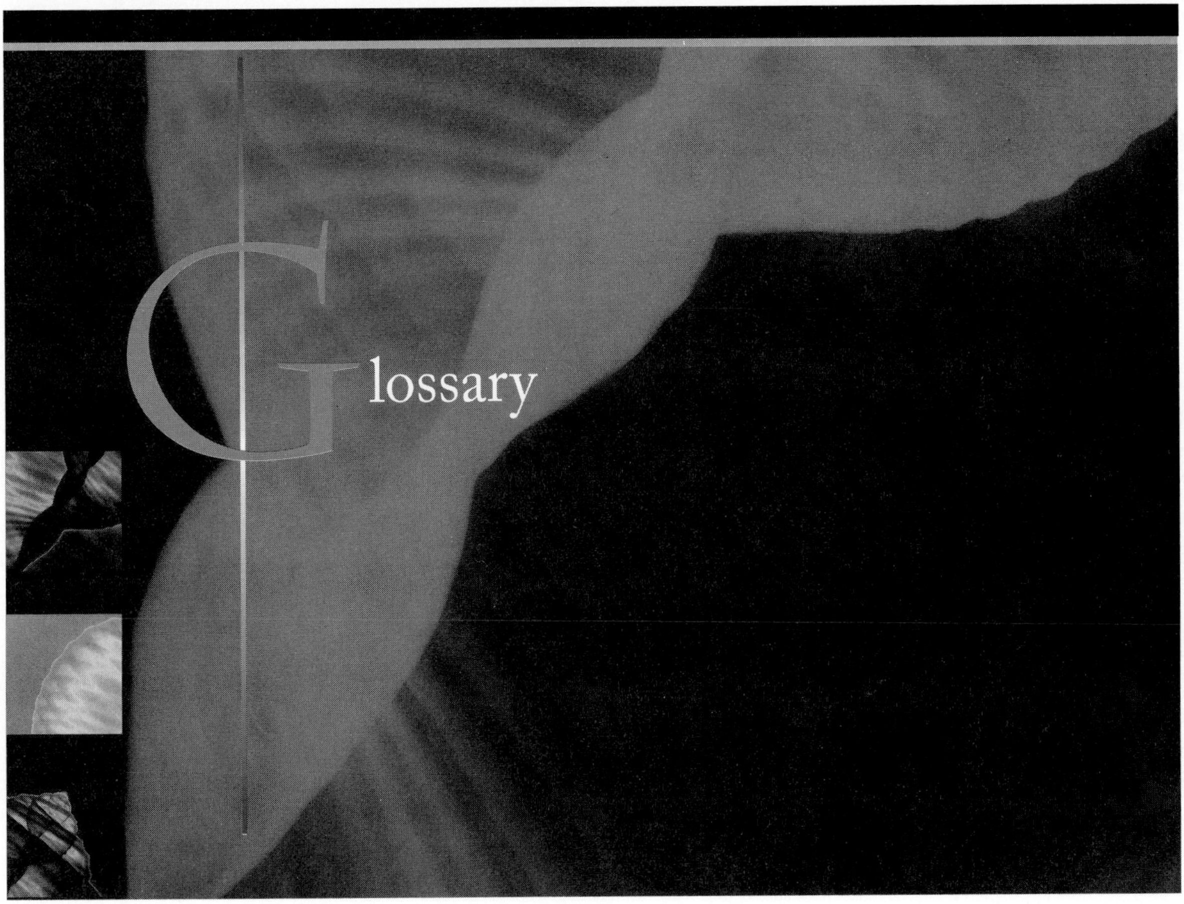

Glossary

abortion Expulsion or removal of a usually nonviable fetus (a fetus that cannot live outside the uterus at that time).

active euthanasia The ending of another person's life by an aggressive method to end suffering.

active suicide The taking of one's own life through a conscious act.

administrative law Law determining the licensing and regulation of the practice of imaging professionals and regulating some employer-employee relations.

advance directive A predetermined (usually written) choice made to inform others of the ways in which the patient wishes to be treated while incompetent. Also a living will that contains written instructions for future health care.

artificial insemination The depositing of seminal fluid within the vagina or cervix by means other than a penis.

assault A deliberate act wherein one person threatens to harm another without consent and the victim feels the attacker has the ability to carry out the threat.

autonomy The concept that patients are to be treated as individuals and informed about procedures to facilitate appropriate decisions.

battery Touching to which the victim has not consented.

beneficience Performance of good acts.

caring A function of the whole person in which concern for the growth and well-being of another is expressed in an integrated application of the mind, body, and spirit that seeks to maximize positive outcomes.

case law Law developed from precedents set during civil and criminal trials.

civil law Law that addresses wrongs committed by one party harming another. Penalties for violation can include monetary damages to compensate for loss and to punish.

collegial model A cooperative method of providing health care for the patient involving sharing, trust, and the pursuit of common goals. This model may be helpful in addressing patients' emotional needs and engaging their cooperation.

common law Law encompassing principles and rules based on ancient usages and customs.

competence The ability to make choices.

complaint The written allegation of wrongdoing filed to initiate a lawsuit. It also may be called a claim or petition, depending on the court in which it is brought.

confidentiality The duty owed by health care providers to protect the privacy of patient information.

consequentialism An ethical school of thought in which decisions are based on the consequences or outcomes of a given act; the good of an activity is evaluated based on whether immediate harm is balanced with future benefits.

consent forms Useful tools to help inform patients about procedures and document consent.

continuous quality control The aspect of quality assurance that monitors technical equipment to maintain quality standards.

contractual model A health care model that defines health care as a business relationship between the provider and patient. A contractual arrangement serves as the guideline for decision making and provision of services.

criminal law
Law that seeks to redress wrongs against the state.

critical thinking
Purposeful, self-regulatory judgment resulting in interpretation, analysis, evaluation, and inference.

cultural values Values specific to a people or culture.

death Cessation of life; lack of biologic function.

defamation The making of a false statement to a third party that is harmful to another's reputation. Defamatory statements may concern patients, family members, visitors, other employees, or physicians.

defendant The party called to answer the allegations made in a lawsuit or criminal case.

deontology An ethical school of thought that bases decision making on individual motives and morals rather than consequences and examines the significance of actions themselves. Deontologic problem solving uses personal rules of right and wrong derived from individual actions, relationships of all kinds, and society.

deposition Oral testimony given under oath during the discovery phase of a trial.

development Ability to grow and continue the life process.

discovery phase The phase of a trial in which attorneys seek to ascertain the truth concerning an incident. During the discovery phase, questions may be asked of any of the parties (including employees and students of a party) either in writing (interrogatories) or orally (depositions). Parties are under oath regardless of whether questions are oral or written. Their statements may be used at trial if testimony contradicts or does not agree with earlier statements.

dismissal The ending of a trial before it goes to the jury; may occur because of lack of evidence or lack of legal grounds to pursue a lawsuit.

diversity Differences rooted in culture, age, experience, health status, gender, sexual orientation, racial or ethnic identity, mental abilities, and other aspects of sociocultural description and socioeconomic status.

documentation Standardized recording of information necessary for continuity of patient care and to protect from medical negligence litigation risks.

due process The notion that persons accused of some infraction have a right to certain paths of recourse. It requires that specific procedures be followed in bringing charges against a person to ensure fairness.

duty to warn third parties The obligation to disclose information to third parties to warn them of a risk of violence, contagious disease, or some other risk.

egalitarian theory Health care distribution theory that demands equal distribution of equal opportunities and resources.

employment at will A policy that allows employers and employees to terminate their relationship for no cause, subject to the restrictions of antidiscrimination and other statutes. The concept of an implied contract provides an exception to the policy, as does the public policy exception.

engineering model A health care model that identifies the health care provider as a scientist concerned with facts and defines the patient as a condition or procedure, not a person. A health care professional using the engineering model tends to view a patient as a collection of body systems, instead of as a whole.

entitlement theory A system of contracts in which a patient has to pay for the contract.

ethics The system or code of conduct and morals advocated by a particular individual or group.

euthanasia Deliberately ending the life of another to end suffering.

existential care Compassion arising from an awareness of common bonds of humanity and common expressions, fates, and feelings.

fairness theory Health care distribution theory that adjusts the equality of individuals with the inequality of their needs and resources.

false imprisonment The unlawful confinement of a person within a fixed area.

health care A practice, a commodity, an approach, or a collective responsibility to ensure the wellness of a population.

hostile work environment sexual harassment Harassment that occurs when sexual behaviors unreasonably interfere with work performance or create an intimidating, hostile, or offensive work environment. Sexual suggestions, sexually derogatory remarks, and sexually motivated physical contact may constitute hostile work environment sexual harassment. Actions of supervisors, co-workers, and customers can give rise to hostile work environment claims. Employers are liable if they create or condone a discriminatory work environment.

inappropriate documentation Recording of opinions or derogatory comments that may result in liability.

informed consent The written assent of a patient to receive a proposed treatment; adequate information is essential for the patient to give truly informed consent.

intentional torts Wrongs resulting from acts done with the intention of causing harm to another.

interrogatory Written testimony given under oath during the discovery phase of a trial.

in vitro fertilization The process by which conception takes place in a laboratory medium.

-isms Prejudgments entailing a tendency to judge others according to a standard considered ideal or presumed to be "normal."

judicial decisions Previous cases that either interpret statutes or adopt and adapt common law principles.

law A body of rules of action or conduct prescribed by controlling authority and having binding legal force. Its basis is in common law from England but has been molded by statutes and judicial decisions since the birth of the United States.

lawsuit A legal action taken in a court for redress of wrongs; it is generally comprised of a pleading phase, discovery phase, and trial.

legislation All the laws and statutes put in place by elected officials in federal, state, city, and county governments.

lie A falsehood told to another who has a reasonable expectation of the truth.

life The entire state of the living thing.

managed care Any type of delivery and reimbursement system that monitors or controls types, quality, use, and costs of health care.

medical indication principle Procedures a physician should follow from a medical point of view after being granted informed consent from the patient to produce more medical good than evil.

medical negligence A breach of the health care provider's obligation to follow the appropriate standard of care that results in harm to the patient.

multiculturalism Respect for the diversity of the many ways of knowing beyond the Western model, brought about by a broadening of learning and an opening of the mind to new ways of thought.

nature of the truth The kind of information expected.

negligence An unintentional tort involving duty, breach of duty, injury, and causation.

no-code order Order not to resuscitate if the patient's heart stops.

nonmaleficence The avoidance of evil.

passive euthanasia The ending of another person's life by withdrawing treatment.

passive suicide The refusal of treatment by a person who knows that refusal will lead to death.

paternalistic (priestly) model A health care model that casts the care giver in the omniscient, paternalistic role of making decisions for patients rather than with patients. Those who subscribe to this model generally believe they know best and tend to discount the patient's feelings.

patient data sheet A uniform document for the recording of pertinent medical information; crucial for adequate risk management.

patient-focused care A health care distribution model that calls for decentralization of patient care services and cross-training of health care professionals.

personal values Beliefs and attitudes held by an individual that provide a foundation for behavior and the way the individual experiences life. Religious convictions, family, political beliefs, education, life experiences, and culture influence personal values.

place of communication The environment of the expectation of truth.

plaintiff The party making the allegations in a lawsuit or criminal case.

pleading phase The phase of a trial in which the plaintiff files a complaint (also called a claim or a petition, depending on the court in which it is brought) against a defendant with the court. The complaint alleges that the plaintiff has been injured as a result of the action or inaction of the defendant. The defendant must file a written answer to the allegations in the complaint.

practical wisdom Right reason or virtue ethics that includes a consideration of emotional factors and development of the reason balanced by consideration of the consequences for the individual in society.

prima facie case of employment discrimination What must be proven by a complainant making a claim of employment discrimination. It requires complainants to prove they belong to a protected class, were qualified for the position, were not hired or were discharged, and after their discharge the employer continued to look for an individual with the complainant's qualifications to fill the position or hired an individual less qualified than the complainant who was not a member of that protected class.

principle of double effect A person may perform an act that has evil effects or risk such effects as long as four certain conditions are met (see page 30).

procedural due proces The mechanism by which individuals can refute attempts by government or other bodies to deprive them of their substantive rights.

professional care The application of the knowledge of a discipline, including its science, theory, practice, and art.

professional values The general attributes prized by a professional group.

professionalism An awareness of the conduct, aims, and qualities defining a given profession, familiarity with professional codes of ethics, and understanding of ethical schools of thought, patient-professional interaction models, and patient rights.

quality assurance A process to assess quality of patient care that uses hospital committees to oversee the quality of various hospital functions.

quality improvement Performing procedures correctly and anticipating, meeting, or exceeding the needs of customers.

quality of life Essential traits that make life worth living.

quid pro quo sexual harassment Harassment that occurs when initial or continued employment or advancement depends on sexual conduct. A supervisor or manager must necessarily be involved in quid pro quo sexual harassment cases.

radiation protection A set of safety procedures involving appropriate radiation protection education, proper equipment maintenance and calibration, quality control and assurance procedures, consistent shielding and collimation, clear policies concerning pregnant patients, and adequate documentation.

rational choice principle A choice made in keeping with the choice most likely to have been made by the patient had the patient been competent.

reasonable care The degree of care a reasonable person, similarly situated, would use.

res ipsa loquitur Latin term meaning "the thing speaks for itself." It is a legal concept invoked in situations in which a particular injury could not have occurred in the absence of negligence.

right A claim or an entitlement.

rights theory Health care distribution theory that claims individuals have a right to health care because of their human dignity and because society has an obligation to serve those needs.

risk management The system for identifying, analyzing, and evaluating risks and selecting the most advantageous method for treating them. Its goal is to maintain quality patient care and conserve the facility's financial resources.

role of communication The relationship between the communicators, which may have an impact on the expectation of truth.

sanctity of human life The ideal underpinning the obligation not to take human life.

secret Knowledge a person has a right or obligation to conceal.

sexual harassment Unwelcome sexual advances, requests for sexual favors, and other verbal and physical conduct of a sexual nature that the employee is required to submit to as a term or condition of employment; the use of submission to or rejection of such conduct as the basis for employment decisions also constitutes sexual harassment, as does behavior having the purpose or effect of unreasonably interfering with work performance or creating an intimidating, hostile, or offensive working environment.

simple consent The assent required of a patient for any procedure.

slippery slope When one act leads to another and then to another at an accelerating rate.

standard of care The degree of skill or care practiced by a reasonable professional practicing in the same field.

statutory duty to report Legal obligation to report a variety of medical conditions and incidents, including venereal disease; contagious diseases such as tuberculosis; wounds inflicted by violence; poisonings; industrial accidents; abortions; drug abuse; and abuse of children, elderly people, and people with disabilities.

statutory law Law including all laws enacted by federal, state, city, and county governments.

substantive due process The notion that the rights of individuals and the circumstances under which those rights may be restricted must be clearly defined and regulated.

suicide The act of knowingly ending one's life.

surrogate A person who substitutes for another, often in decision-making processes.

terminal illness A condition that leaves the patient irreversibly comatose or will lead to death within a year.

tort A subdivision of civil law under which actions are filed to recover damages for personal injury or property damage occurring from negligent conduct or intentional misconduct. The types of torts most likely to be encountered by imaging professionals include assault, battery, false imprisonment, defamation, negligence, lack of informed consent, and breach of patient confidentiality.

triage A system of prioritizing that encourages the routing of treatment to those with the greatest opportunity for a positive outcome.

trial The part of a lawsuit in which the facts of a case are presented to a judge or jury for a decision.

truthfulnes Conformity with fact or reality.

unintentional torts Wrongs resulting from actions that were not intended to do harm.

utilitarian theory Health care distribution theory that calls for realizing the greatest good for the greatest number.

values Qualities or standards desirable or worthy of esteem in themselves; they are expressed in behaviors, language, and standards of conduct.

veracity The obligation to tell the truth and not to lie or deceive others.

virtue ethics A new ethical school of thought that focuses on the use of practical wisdom for emotional and intellectual problem solving. It incorporates elements of teleology and deontology to provide a more holistic approach to solving ethical dilemmas.

APPENDIX A

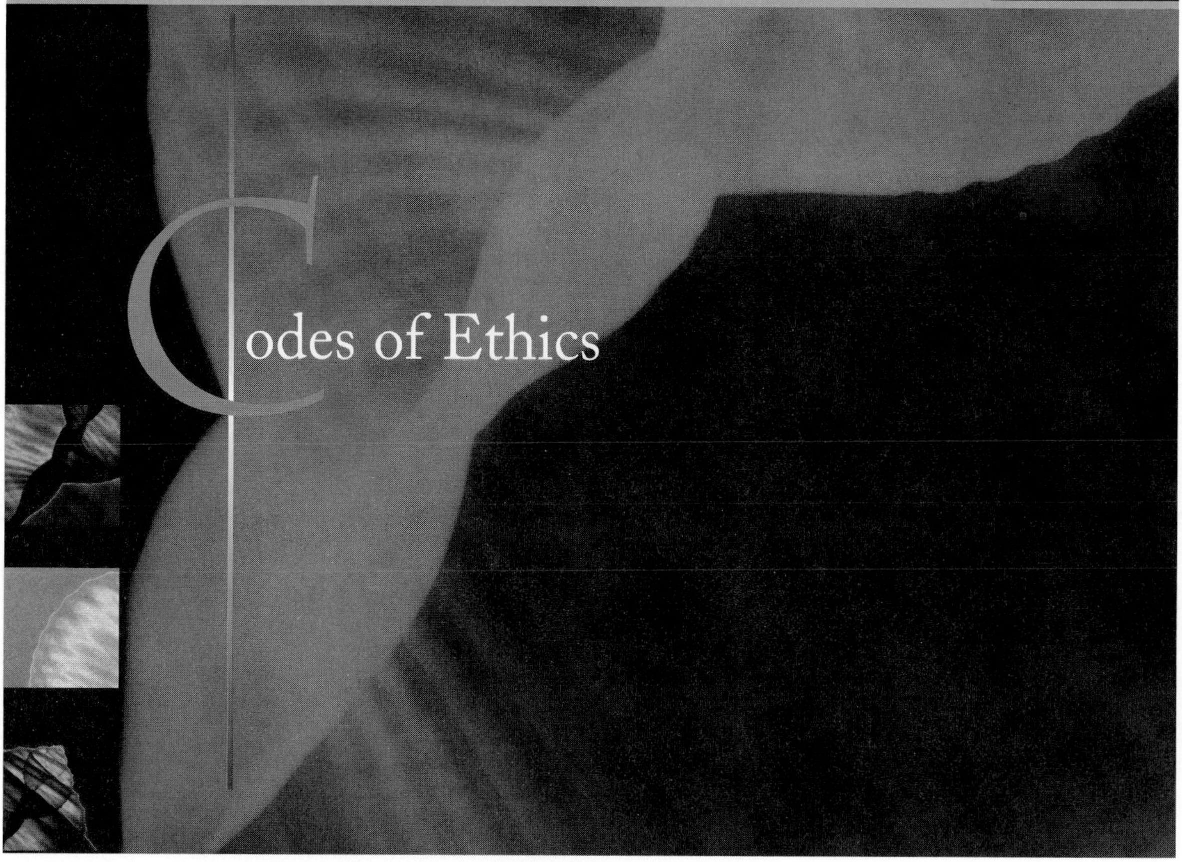

Codes of Ethics

APPENDIX OUTLINE

AMERICAN SOCIETY OF RADIOLOGIC TECHNOLOGISTS AND THE AMERICAN REGISTRY OF RADIOLOGIC TECHNOLOGISTS CODE OF ETHICS

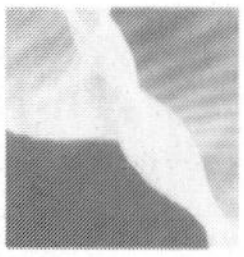

1. The radiologic technologist conducts himself or herself in a professional manner, responds to patient needs and supports colleagues and associates in providing quality patient care.
2. The radiologic technologist acts to advance the principal objective of the profession to provide services to humanity with full respect for the dignity of mankind.
3. The radiologic technologist delivers patient care and service unrestricted by concerns of personal attributes or the nature of the disease or illness, and without discrimination, regardless of sex, race, creed, religion or socioeconomic status.
4. The radiologic technologist practices technology founded upon theoretical knowledge and concepts, utilizes equipment and accessories consistent with the purpose for which they have been designed, and employs procedures and techniques appropriately.
5. The radiologic technologist assesses situations, exercises care, discretion and judgment, assumes responsibility for professional decisions, and acts in the best interest of the patient.
6. The radiologic technologist acts as an agent through observation and communication to obtain pertinent information for the physician to aid in the diagnosis and treatment management of the patient, and recognizes the interpretation and diagnosis are outside the scope of practice for the profession.
7. The radiologic technologist utilizes equipment and accessories, employs techniques and procedures, performs services in accordance with an accepted standard of practice and demonstrates expertise in minimizing the radiation exposure to the patient, self and other members of the health care team.
8. The radiologic technologist practices ethical conduct appropriate to the profession and protects the patient's right to quality radiologic technology care.
9. The radiologic technologist respects confidences entrusted in the course of professional practice, respects the patient's right to privacy and reveals confidential information only as required by law or to protect the welfare of the individual or the community.
10. The radiologic technologist continually strives to improve knowledge and skills by participating in educational and professional activities, sharing knowledge with colleagues and investigating new and innovative aspects of professional practice. One means available to improve knowledge and skills is through professional continuing education.

Revised and adopted by The American Society of Radiologic technologists and The American Registry of Radiologic Technologists, Albuquerque, NM, July 1994.

CODE OF ETHICS FOR THE PROFESSION OF DIAGNOSTIC MEDICAL ULTRASOUND

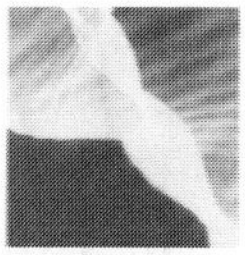

PREAMBLE

The goal of this code of ethics is to promote excellence in patient care by fostering responsibility and accountability and thereby help to ensure the integrity of professionals involved in all aspects of diagnostic medical ultrasound.

OBJECTIVES

- To create an environment where professional and ethical issues are discussed
- To help the individual practitioner identify ethical issues
- To provide guidelines for individual practitioners regarding ethical behavior

PRINCIPLES

Principle I: In order to promote patient well-being, professionals shall:

A. Provide information about the procedure and the reason it is being done. Respond to patient's concerns and questions.
B. Respect the patient's self-determination and the right to refuse the procedure.
C. Recognize the patient's individuality and provide care in a non-judgmental and non-discriminatory manner.
D. Promote the privacy, dignity and comfort of the patient and his/her family.
E. Protect the confidentiality of acquired patient information.
F. Strive to ensure patient safety.

Principle II: To promote the highest level of competent practice, professionals shall:

A. Obtain the appropriate education and skills to ensure competence.
B. Practice according to published and recognized standards.
C. Work to achieve and maintain appropriate credentials.
D. Acknowledge personal limits and not practice beyond their capacity and skills.
E. Perform only those procedures that are medically indicated, restricting practice to validated and appropriate tests. For research studies, follow established research protocol, obtaining (and documenting) informed patient consent as needed.
F. Ensure the completeness of examinations and the timely communication of important information.
G. Strive for excellence and continued competence through continuing education.
H. Perform ongoing quality assurance.
I. NOT compromise patient care by the use of substances that may alter judgment or skill.

Principle III. To promote professional integrity and public trust, the professional shall:

A. Be truthful and promote honesty in interactions with patients, colleagues and the public.
B. Accurately represent their level of competence, education and certification.
C. Avoid situations which may constitute a conflict of interest.
D. Maintain appropriate personal boundaries with patients including avoidance of inappropriate conduct, be it verbal or nonverbal.
E. Promote cooperative relationships within the profession and with other members of the health care community.
F. Avoid situations which exploit others for financial gain or misrepresent information to obtain reimbursement.
G. Promote equitable access to care.

Courtesy Society of Diagnostic Medical Sonographers, Dallas, Texas.

AMERICAN SOCIETY OF RADIOLOGIC TECHNOLOGISTS RADIATION THERAPIST CODE OF ETHICS

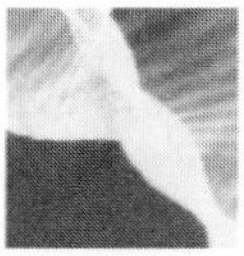

1. The radiation therapist advances the principal objective of the profession to provide services to humanity with full respect for the dignity of mankind.
2. The radiation therapist delivers patient care and service unrestricted by concerns of personal attributes or the nature of the disease or illness, and non-discriminatory with respect to race, color, creed, sex, age, disability or national origin.
3. The radiation therapist assesses situations; exercises care, discretion and judgment; assumes responsibility for professional decisions; and acts in the best interest of the patient.
4. The radiation therapist adheres to the tenets and domains of the scope of practice for radiation therapists.
5. The radiation therapist actively engages in lifelong learning to maintain, improve and enhance professional competence and knowledge.

Revised and adopted by The American Society of Radiologic Technologists and The American Registry of Radiologic Technologists, July 1994.

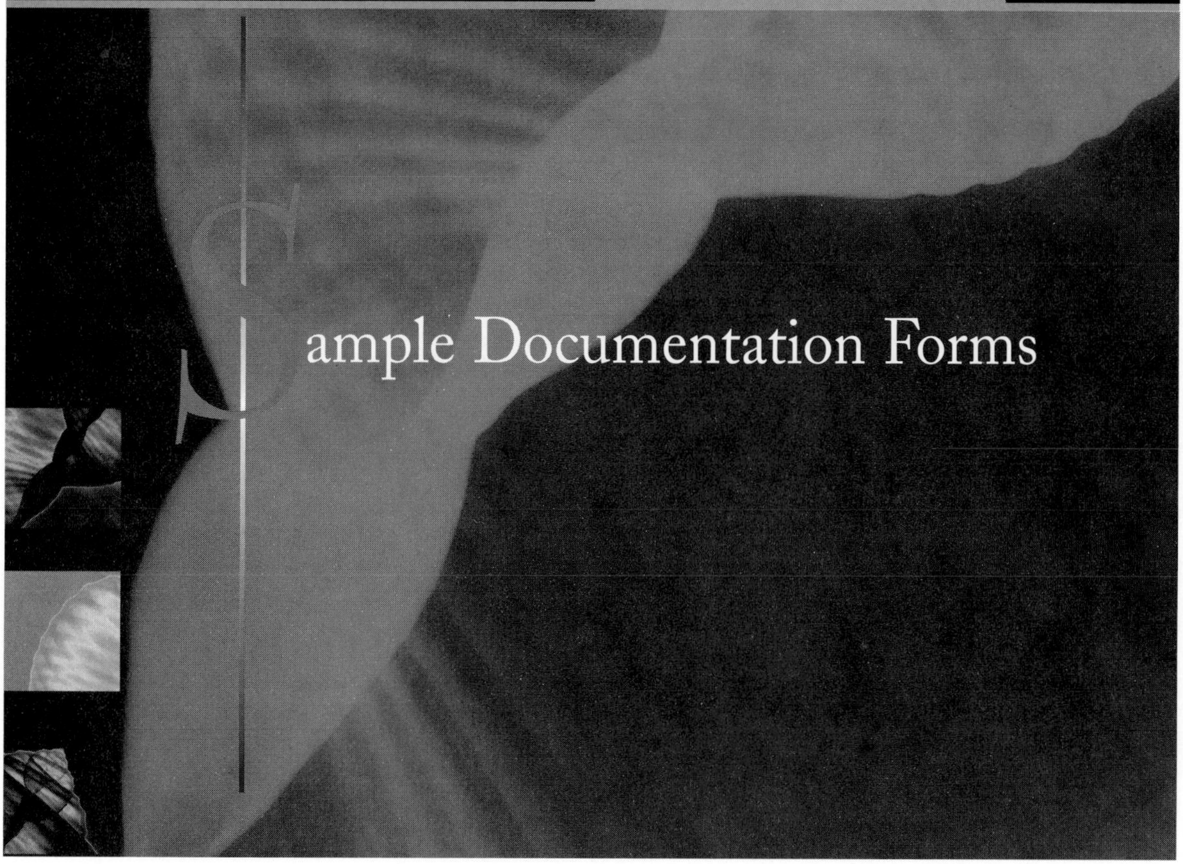

Sample Documentation Forms

PATIENT/VISITOR: UNUSUAL INCIDENT, MEDICATION ERROR & ACCIDENT REPORT	**VISITOR INFORMATION:** Name: Address: Patient Visited:	**PATIENT INFORMATION:** Location: Name: Hospital #: Inpatient ______ Outpatient _______ IF NOT IMPRINTED, PLEASE PRINT HOSP. NO., NAME, DATE AND LOCATION

I. **DESCRIPTION OF INCIDENT:** check *all* that apply; (if other, specify)

A. Location: (specify unit) ________________________ Date: __________________ Time: ________________

B) **Insult/Injury to Tissue/Skin**
___Abrasion
___Bruise
___Burn
___IV Infiltration
___Laceration
___Pressure Area
___Puncture
___Other (specify)_____

C) **Med/IV**
___Duplication
___Omission
___Transcription Error
___Wrong Dose/Rate
___Wrong Med
___Wrong Patient
___Wrong Solution
___Wrong Route
___Wrong Time
___Other (specify)_____

D) ___**Fall**
___Fall Precautions in Place
___Siderails Up
___Siderails Down
Location:______________
Activity:______________
Mental Status/Orientation:
____

E) **Equipment/Device Related** (specify)________________

F) **Miscellaneous**
___Accident (specify)
___Delayed/Cancelled Test/Procedure
___Missing/Damaged Property
___Other (specify)_______

II. **BRIEF NARRATIVE:**____

MED/IV: Identify the total amount of incorrect medication or IV fluid and the number of dosages the patient received.

Immediate Action Taken: ____

Physician Notification Necessary: Yes____ N.A.____ Name of Physician:__________________ Date:________ Time:______

Name of Witness/Observer: (if applicable)____

Work Unit/Address:____

Immediate Supervisor Notified: Yes____ N.A.____ Name of Supervisor:__________________ Date:________ Time:______

Safety and Security Notified: Yes____ N.A.____ Patient Representatives Notified: Yes____ N.A.____

Signature/Title of Person Completing Report:______________________________ Date:________ Time:______

III. **PHYSICIAN'S REPORT:** (If indicated) (Complete within 24 hours)

Findings/Treatment Related to Incident: ____

Physician's Signature:____ Date:________ Time:______

IV. **FOLLOW UP:** ____

Reviewed by:____ Date:________ Time:______
(Supervisory Signature)

PATIENT DATA SHEET/
PHYSICIAN ORDER FOR
RADIOLOGIC/NUCLEAR MEDICINE
Consultation/Request for Procedure
Department of Radiology

• DO NOT SEND BOTH COPIES OF REQUISITION TO RADIOLOGY.
RETAIN WHITE COPY TO FILE IN PATIENT'S MEDICAL RECORD •

DATE:
HOSP. NO:
NAME:
BIRTHDATE:
ADDRESS:
SS #:

IF NOT IMPRINTED, PLEASE PRINT DATE, HOSP. NO., NAME AND LOCATION

Procedure
Scheduled for Date__________ Time____________
Known Allergies____________________________
Female of Child-Bearing Age ☐ Yes ☐ No **Pregnant** ☐ Yes ☐ No **Lactating** ☐ Yes ☐ No
Isolation ☐ Strict ☐ Respiratory ☐ Protective
☐ Wound/Skin ☐ Enteric ☐ Blood ☐ Secretion/Excretion

Patient
Transport ☐ Walk ☐ Cart ☐ Chair ☐ Isolette
Oxygen ☐ Yes ☐ No **Diabetic** ☐ Yes ☐ No

☐ **Routine** ☐ **ASAP** ☐ **STAT** ☐ **Portable**
STAT Report ☐ Yes ☐ No

Procedure(s)____

Clinical Findings/Relevant Diagnosis:________________________________

Reason for Exam:____

Return films with patient
☐ Yes
☐ No
______CLP No.

Physician Name (print)____________________________ Pager____________

Signature__________________ CLP No.________ Date_______ Clinic/ Unit________ Phone____________

Radiology use only

14×17
11×14
10×12
8×10
9×9
6×12

	KV	MAS	DIST
PA			
LAT			

Fluoro Time (min)__________ Actual Date of Proc.____________
Room__________ Actual Time of Proc.____________
Procedure________________________________
Physician__________________ Technologist/ Sonographer __________
Notes____________________________________

Contrast____________________ Date__________

PHARMACEUTICALS AND AGENTS
Radiopharmaceutical Administered__________________ Amount______ Time______ By______
Route of Administration ☐ I.V. ☐ Oral Other________________ Lot No.__________

Other Agents Administered__________________ Amount______ Time______ By______
Route of Administration ☐ I.V. ☐ Oral Other________________ Lot No.__________

IMAGING INSTRUCTIONS____________________________________

PHYSICIAN'S RADIOPHARMACEUTICAL/
ADJUNCT DRUG PRESCRIPTIONS

☐ **Outpatient** ☐ **Inpatient**

Technologist's Signature ________________________

ANSWERS TO CHAPTER REVIEW QUESTIONS

CHAPTER 1

1. e
2. d
3. a
4. d
5. personal study and investigations, system of professional conduct
6. contractual
7. priestly
8. covenant
9. personal, cultural and professional
10. What is the context in which the ethical problem occurred? What is the significance of the values involved in the problem? What is the meaning of the problem for all the parties involved? What should be done to remedy the problem?
11. d
12. c
13. d
14. c
15. d
16. d
17. d
18. b
19. True
20. True
21. False
22. True
23. False
24. True
25. False
26. True
27. False
28. False
29. True
30. False
31. False

CHAPTER 2

1. d
2. b
3. c
4. nonmaleficence, beneficence
5. a. Action must be good or morally indifferent in itself
   b. Agent must intend only the good effect and not the evil effect
   c. Evil effect cannot be a means to the good effect
   d. Proportionality must exist between good and evil effects.
6. True
7. patient
8. beneficence and nonmaleficence
9. Differences should include the active nature of beneficence and the passive nature of avoidance involved in nonmaleficence, as well as the greater importance of nonmaleficence compared with beneficence.
10. acts involving doing good and avoiding harm
11. avoiding harm
12. education/gathering information and their own input and decision making (among other answers)

13. the degree of skill or care employed by a reasonable professional practicing in the same field
14. scope of practice, educational requirements, and curricula
15. through expert testimony
16. yes
17. duty, breach of duty, injury, and causation
18. an applicable standard of care, deviation from that standard of care, injury and causation
19. yes
20. to provide information to facilitate quality patient care and to minimize litigation risks
21. by providing a written record of what actually transpired
22. consistently following radiation safety and safety policies and procedures
23. True
24. False

CHAPTER 3

1. d
2. diagnosis
   treatment prognosis
   risks
   alternatives
   costs
   rules
   duration of incapacitation
   names of person performing procedure
3. feedback to ensure the patient's understanding of the procedure and opportunity to question
4. the imaging professional may have a limited role in the informed consent process but it is the physician's duty to provide the information about the procedure for informed consent
5. competence—the ability to make decisions concerning one's life
   Surrogacy—the appointment of a person to make decisions for another
6. b
7. a prerogative invoked in limited circumstanced when health care providers withhold information from a patient because they believe the information would have adverse effects on the patient's condition or health
8. a. The patient must be incapable of giving consent and no lawful surrogate is available.
   b. Danger to life or a risk of serious impairment to health is apparent.
   c. Immediate treatment is necessary to avert these dangers.
9. True
10. True
11. False (If the patient perceives the act was intentional, determination of intent could be left to jury)
12. True
13. False
14. False (Only if justified according to conditions in text)
15. True
16. False (The physician has legal duty although imaging professional has duty to ensure consent is obtained)
17. False
18. False (see #16)
19. False

CHAPTER 4

1. conformance with fact or reality
2. place of communication, roles of the communicators, nature of the truth involved
3. practical needs
4. right to the truth
5. confidentiality
6. natural secrets, promised secrets, and professional secrets
7. professional secret
8. mechanisms for reporting certain types of wounds, communicable diseases, auto accidents, birth defects, drug addition, and industrial accidents
9. when the life or safety of a patient is endangered when intervention can prevent threatened suicide or self-injury, or when an innocent third party may be harmed such as abuse situations
10. e
11. False
12. True
13. False
14. False (there are exceptions, although they are rare)
15. True
16. True
17. True
18. False
19. False
20. True
21. False
22. False
23. False
24. False
25. False
26. False

CHAPTER 5

1. entire state
2. life life cycle
3. a. religious reasons
   b. life is the greatest of goods and should be protected
   c. harm to the community
4. a good death, painless death—mercy killing
5. the advanced directive and living wills let the health care provider know the desires of the patient
6. Persistent vegetative state is when the brain stem continues to function, the body is not dead, patient seems to be awake but has no awarenesses of self or environment.
7. a. biologic functions
   b. intellect
   c. emotions, also creativity, contact with others, and needs
8. Active suicide is when the person takes his own life by inflicting the fatal blow and active euthanasia takes place when another inflicts the final blow (mercy killing). They may each present themselves when a person is suffering and believes death will bring relief from that suffering for themselves or for others involved in their suffering.
9. Patients' rights may be carried out through advanced directives, including Do Not Resuscitate Orders, living wills, and durable powers of attorney.
10. The imaging professional must always have consent to perform any diagnostic or therapeutic procedure. If the patient refuses, the imaging professional must respect their wishes.
11. When the patient refuses treatment knowing it will lead to death.
12. true, ethical and legal right to refuse treatment
13. False
14. False. However, physician-assisted suicide may be legal in Oregon at this time.
15. True. If a patient must consent to treatment, that patient can also refuse it.
16. False. It was not articulated in court until 1984.
17. False. Different tests exist, but no definite rules.
18. False. Statutes vary, many stating only competent adults may execute living wills.
19. True. Many statutes exclude the withdrawal of nutrition and hydration.
20. False. Living wills do not require as formal an execution.
21. False. They are protected from liability for carrying out the wishes in a living will.
22. True
23. True. They create a substitute decision maker instead of a specific decision.
24. False. Anyone can be named as the decision maker in a durable power of attorney and is usually a family member.
25. True
26. False. By appointing a decision maker, they apply to all health care decisions when the principal is incompetent.
27. False
28. False
29. False

CHAPTER 6

1. practice, an approach, commodity, or a collective responsibility
2. expensive and scarce
3. a. egalitarian
   b. entitlement
   c. fairness
   d. utilitarian
4. professional identity.
5. a. improved efficiency
   b. empowerment of employees
   c. sensible delegation of duties
   d. better scheduling
   e. cross-training
   f. wise application of automation
6. True
7. False
8. True
9. False
10. True
11. False. They are held to the standard of care of one trained in that area.
12. True
13. False. The imaging professional can be proactive through voluntary cross training, self evaluation and waste reduction.
14. False. Generally. Although it would seem they should be, federal law generally prevents suits against HMO. State legislatures are trying to change this but to date, Texas is the only state which has done so.
15. True. The Wickline case suggests that physicians must fight the denial of treatment by third party payors.
16. True. Particularly in outpatient situations when the imaging professional is the person dealing with patient, ordering physician and interpreting physician.
17. True. Particularly in outpatient situations when the imaging professional is the person dealing with patient, ordering physician and interpreting physician. The imaging professional may have an obligation to make the involved physician aware of the severity of the patient's symptoms.

CHAPTER 7

1. students and programs
2. ethical theories
3. contract and covenant
4. d
5. truthfulness and confidentiality
6. justice
7. a worthwhile quality—a value
8. JRC and ARRT
9. [short essay]
10. the Fourteenth Amendment to the United States Constitution
11. substantive due process, which defines and regulates the rights of citizens and the circumstances when those rights may be restricted; procedural due process, which provides an opportunity to refute attempts to deprive citizens of their substantive rights.
12. 1. a written statement regarding the reasons for the proposed action, 2. formal notice of a hearing where the student may answer the charges, and 3. a hearing at which both sides may present their case and any rebuttal evidence
13. employment at will, which means that either employer or employee may terminate their relationship at any time for no cause, subject to antidiscrimination or other statutes
14. implied contract exception, public policy exception
15. True
16. False. Parties can agree to almost anything as long as both parties know to what they are agreeing. What they are getting unless the parties are contract is grossly unfair. An exception is when the bargaining power of the parties is greatly mismatched and the contract is grossly unfair to the party with less bargaining power.
17. True
18. False
19. False. Students have due process rights. First, it must be determined whether a student's substantive rights have been denied. If so, they are entitled to at least the following: 1. A written statement regarding the reasons for the proposed action, 2. Formal notice of a hearing where the student may answer the charges, and 3. A hearing at which both sides may present their case and any rebuttal evidence
20. True
21. False. Substantive rights must be denied before procedural due process rights come into play.
22. False. Students have due process rights. First, it must be determined whether a student's substantive rights have been denied. If so, they are entitled to at least the following: 1. A written statement regarding the reasons for the proposed action, 2. Formal notice of a hearing where the student may answer the charges, and 3. A hearing at which both sides may present their case and any rebuttal evidence.
23. True
24. False. They should be published in handbooks or institutional regulations.
25. False. The hearing committe should be unbiased.
26. False. A student has the right to remain silent without it being used against him or her.
27. True
28. False. Only evidence presented at the hearing may be considered.
29. False. The student is entitled to an appeal.
30. False. Employment is generally governed by the employment at will doctrine with restrictions by antidiscrimination and other statutes.
31. False. Under the employment at will doctrine either employer or employee may terminate their relationship at any time for no cause, subject to antidiscrimination or other statutes.

CHAPTER 8

1. the differences that may be rooted in culture, age, experience, health status, gender, sexual orientation, racial identity, mental abilities, and other aspects of sociocultural organization and socioeconomic position
2. adaptation of resources for people of all backgrounds
3. physical and mental health, sexual orientation, age, ethnicity and gender
4. income marital status, geographic location, education and religion
5. interaction patterns
6. at the beginning of the program and through the program
7. to better understand better patients differing reactions to the imaging environment, the way patients make choices, and the need to employ ethical decision making and provide a variety of ways to help patients understand procedures
8. language courses, visual aids interpreters, patient advocates, and informational sessions—continuing education
9. race, gender, age, national origin, religion, or disability
10. the ARRT and ASRT codes of ethics (see appendix A)

11. employment situations
12. disparate treatment
13. disparate impact
14. 1. the complainant belongs to a protected group
    2. the complainant was qualified for the position
    3. despite the qualifications, the complainant was not hired or was discharged
    4. the employer continued to look for an individual with the complainant's qualifications to fill the position or hired an individual less qualified than the complainant who was not a member of that protected class
15. sexual harassment claims
16. quid pro quo
17. hostile work environment
18. 1. The employee must be a member of a protected class.
    2. The employee must have been subject to unwelcome sexual harassment in the form of sexual advances, requests for sexual favors, or other verbal or physical conduct of a sexual nature.
    3. The complained of conduct must have been based on gender.
    4. The conduct must have had the effect of unreasonably interfering with the employee's work performance and creating a working environment a reasonable person would find intimidating, hostile, abusive, or offensive and the employee perceived as abusive.
    5. The employer knew or should have known of the harassment and failed to take appropriate action.
19. If the HIV infected or AIDS patients are seen as a "direct threat" to the health and safety of others. "Direct threat" is defined as a significant risk that cannot be eliminated by a modification of policies, practices, or procedures, or by the provision of auxiliary aids or services.
20. True
21. False
22. True
23. False
24. False
25. False
26. False

CHAPTER 9

1. the function in which a person expresses concern for the growth and well being of another in an integrated application of the mind, body, and spirit designed to maximize positive outcomes
2. professional caring is characterized by the application of the knowledge of a professional discipline, including its science, theory, practice, and art
3. compassion arising from an awareness of common bonds of humanity and common expressions, fates, and feelings
4. human caring
5. ideal
6. scarcity of time technical priorities impact of personal life, lack of training in caring for critically ill and terminal patients, lack of communication, societal pressures, lack of faith in oneself
7. individual and institutional

8-9. [short essay]

10. True
11. False
12. True
13. True
14. False
15. True
16. True
17. True
18. False
19. False
20. False. Eight times as many patients suffer injuries from negligence as file malpractice suits.
21. True. Patients generally do not consult an attorney unless they are dissatisfied with the "care" they receive.

CHAPTER 10

1. D
2. organ donor and the recipient

3-6. [short essay]

7. True
8. False
9. False. The law is still evolving, particularly because reproductive methods are ever changing.
10. False. Although legislators try to anticipate what effect technology will have, the laws are generally written after the problems arise.
11. True
12. True

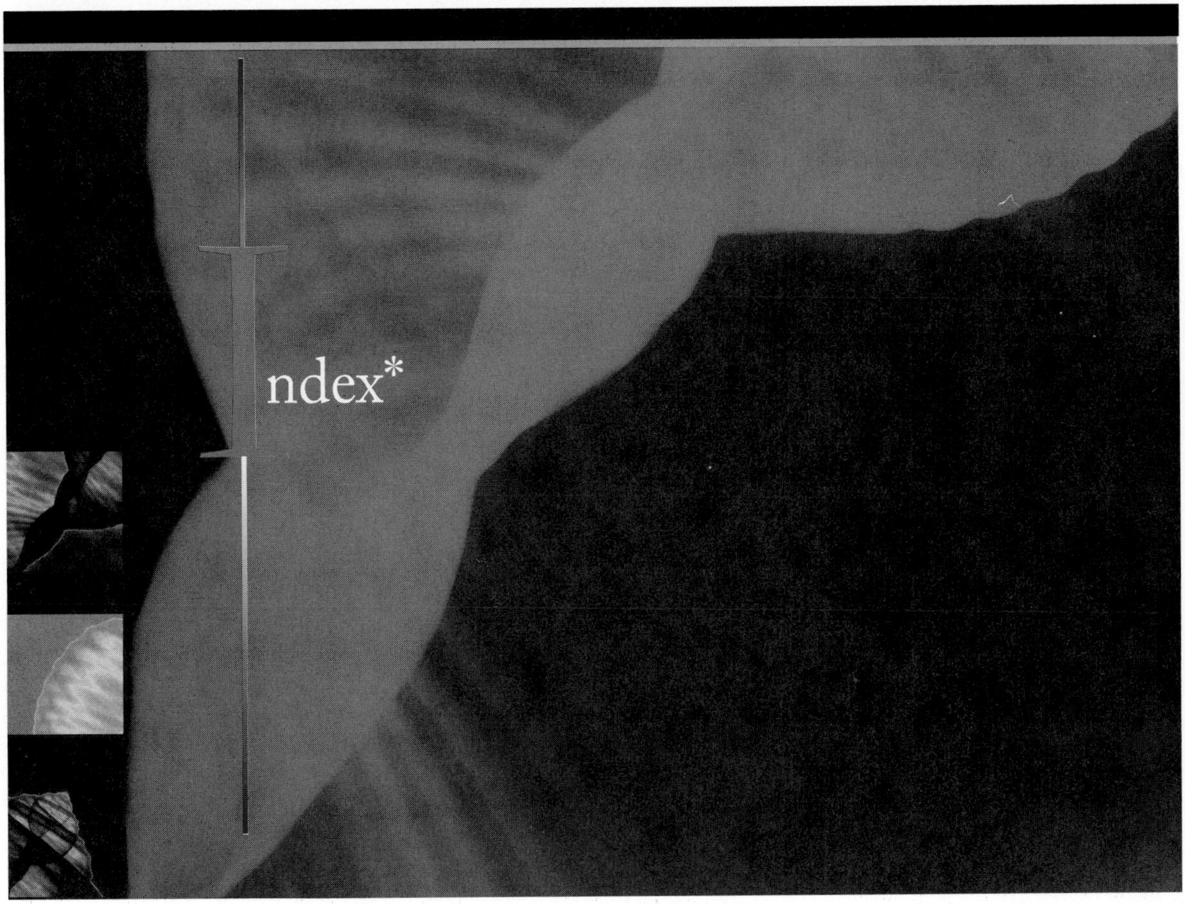

Index*

*Page numbers in italics indicate illustrations and boxes; *t* indicates tables.

A

F

Q

R